Activities of Daily Living
—an ADL Guide for
Alzheimer's Care—

by Kathy Laurenhue, M.A.

Published by: Wiser Now, Inc.   800-999-0795

www.wisernow.com
Write or call for information on purchasing copies in bulk.

ISBN 0-9786362-1-X

Wiser Now, Inc.
11949 Whistling Way
Bradenton, FL 34202
800-999-0795
Kathy@wisernow.com

See also the companion book to this one:
Alzheimer's Basic Caregiving – an ABC Guide

This book is dedicated to my beloved mother

who tried to teach me that

even when life is most demanding—

indeed, perhaps especially then—

"Joy is all around you. Let it find you."

Table of Contents

I ntroduction

No one in our family ever suffered from insanity.
We've always enjoyed it.
—*Author Unknown*

For all the years that my mother had Alzheimer's disease (AD), I kept that plaque on my desk as a reminder that laughter is still the best medicine. I certainly wasn't always successful at keeping the demons of anger, guilt and sorrow at bay, but many years after my mother's death, I am still grateful for the gifts within the grief – the lemonade potential within the lemons, if you will.

This book is intended to be a highly practical and not entirely serious look at managing the basic caregiving needs called ADLs or Activities of Daily Living (dressing, bathing, grooming, etc.) of people with Alzheimer's disease and related forms of dementia. AD is a terrible disease, but you won't survive the caregiving years if you don't keep your sense of humor, find the absurd within the awful, and awaken your curiosity over the odd ways the brain works.

I have been writing about Alzheimer's disease for 15 years now. I have developed hundreds of hours of curriculum for national long-term care companies throughout the U.S. and Australia, and for multi-media training companies and the National Alzheimer's Association. Yet one of the most rewarding things I've done was produce an international, award-winning newsletter for caregivers of people with Alzheimer's disease. This book and its companion, *Alzheimer's Basic Caregiving – an ABC Guide*, are outgrowths of those 4-page monthly compositions.

What this book isn't: There are a great many ethical, financial and legal concerns that need to be addressed when someone has dementia. There are complex decisions to make about support services and who will provide care where. I am also a strong believer in meaningful occupation of people with dementia. In order to limit the length of this book, I have not addressed any of those topics here, but I have written about them in other formats, and may produce sequels. See also the Resources and Bibliography at the end of this book.

One caution: People with Alzheimer's disease remain unique individuals. What works for one person may not work for another. What works today, may not work tomorrow and what didn't work yesterday may work today. There are no single right answers. Experiment. Try new approaches.

And **one disclaimer:** I am not a doctor or a nurse; nothing suggested on these pages is meant to substitute for medical supervision by qualified professionals. I've tried to provide accurate explanations and useful advice based on what is currently known about Alzheimer's disease, but new research and deeper understanding may invalidate what is stated here.

Activities of daily living

A few words about terminology

As the opening quote in the introduction might indicate, I don't believe in using words like "suffer" or "victim". There is tragedy in every human life; using a word like "victim" sets the other person apart and makes him an object of pity, as if we are not equal in our humanity. Such words also seem to be at odds with words like "hope" and "joy," which can still be a vital part of the lives of both caregiver and care receiver. In this book I want to share what I know about how we can connect with one another, no matter what our varying disabilities may be. What I learned from my mother and countless others with dementia is that everyone – *everyone* – has something to share if we are only open to their gifts.

On a more mundane note:

- I have tried to avoid saying "he or she" by simply alternating among the pronouns and hope that doesn't cause confusion.
- I have tended to use "dementia" and "Alzheimer's disease" (AD) interchangeably because AD is the most common form of dementia. I hope *that* doesn't cause confusion.
- Although it is sometimes awkward, I have steadfastly used the words "person with dementia" or "people with Alzheimer's disease," because the condition is always secondary to the individual. Sometimes I have just used "person" and hope that "with AD" is understood. At other times I've used "care receiver," but the goal is always to build a relationship in which the care flows both ways.
- "Caregiver" is usually used to indicate both family members and professionals. I recognize that the physical and emotional circumstances in which they are

giving care are often quite different, but both families and professionals need the same understanding of the person who has dementia and what the condition has done to his brain. When I want to refer particularly to the relationship between family members, I often refer to the care receiver as a "loved one" even though it sounds like a funeral director speaking of the "dearly departed." Sometimes I find the English language woefully inadequate.

- **Ain't Misbehavin'** – When I was first "getting into" Alzheimer's disease, all the resources I found were negative and depressing, and it seemed to me, people with AD were constantly being faulted for behavior that was being portrayed as aberrant and bizarre. I saw things differently. People with AD were trying to communicate. I began a monthly newsletter column called "Ain't Misbehavin'" (after the Broadway show) to try to interpret their messages. I have continued to use that term in many of the chapters of this book.

My basic tenets

Here are my immutable tenets for providing quality care to someone with Alzheimer's disease.

1. If you've met one person with Alzheimer's disease, you've met one person with Alzheimer's disease. People with AD (and related forms of dementia) may have a common condition, but they remain unique individuals, and the course of their disease is never entirely predictable.

2. Always treat the individual first, the condition second. It is more important to know the individual than the disease. (But knowing the disease is helpful, too.)

3. Fear is the most pervasive negative emotion in people with AD. It's up to us to make them feel safe and secure.

4. Pain is the most commonly undiagnosed condition in people with AD because they lose the ability to verbalize their discomfort. Look daily for nonverbal signs of pain, and check with a doctor about relieving it.

5. The person with Alzheimer's disease cannot control the progression of the disease in his body. Therefore it is up to us to adapt our care to his needs.

6. People with Alzheimer's disease retain the full range of human emotions and deserve to be treated as our equals – always with dignity, but rarely with solemnity. Sharing our sense of humor is a great equalizer.

7. People with dementia lose brain cells. They do not lose their desire to feel useful and valued. They still have gifts to contribute.

8. People with Alzheimer's disease always make sense to themselves. It's up to us to decipher their messages.

9. You will never win an argument with someone with Alzheimer's disease.

10. People with Alzheimer's disease always understand more than they can express, and they are usually excellent at "reading" nonverbal communication and sensing the emotional atmosphere.

11. People with dementia will always stay where they feel they belong. It's up to us to make them comfortable in their surroundings or to remove them to a more reassuring place.

12. The person with Alzheimer's disease is not deliberately trying to upset us. If he were, he would have a different diagnosis.

13. Always assume the person with AD is doing the best he can in any given situation.

14. When a person is willfully resistive, always look for the big five:
    a) fatigue
    b) frustration
    c) fear and confusion
    d) physiological discomfort
    e) environmental agitators.

15. People with Alzheimer's disease may not remember names, but they always know who loves them and whom they love.

  Activities of daily living

1 —Reasons to resist care

Resistance is thought transformed into feeling.
Change the thought that creates the resistance,
and there is no more resistance.
—Robert Conklin

One of the most common laments of both family and professional caregivers is, *I was just trying to help.* Because we enter into each caregiving task with the best of intentions, we are often flabbergasted when a person with Alzheimer's disease resists our care. A hefty portion of the companion book, *Alzheimer's Basic Caregiving – an ABC Guide,* is devoted to the proposition that all behavior is communication; it's up to us to decipher the message. The chief message when someone resists our care is: *I'm uncomfortable.* The potential reasons for the discomfort are many, but most stem from the damage to the brain that dementia causes, and the fear and physical or emotional pain the person is experiencing.

Be aware of changes in the brain

People with Alzheimer's disease often have aphasia, which can mean they don't know *how to say* what they want (expressive aphasia) or *how to interpret* what you have said (receptive aphasia). They may also have apraxia and agnosia, meaning they don't remember how to do common things and they don't recognize common objects. These deficits are compounded by other changes in the brain which mean they may have trouble with the following:

- Getting started or initiating any action – they may need one or many "jump starts"
- Putting the required steps in logical order
- Tapping into the visual spatial senses required for the task

The common causes

When a person resists our assistance, here are some of the common logical reasons for doing so:

Frustration over inability to handle what was once easy
A person may be upset because she *needs* help, whether the disability is:

- a chronic condition such as arthritis that makes the task painful
- memory impairment causing confusion over the mechanics of the task
- a vision deficit that prevents her from clearly seeing what she is doing (such as buttoning a blouse correctly)
- or a hearing deficit which causes her to misinterpret directions.

Physical pain
Arthritis, bursitis, stiff joints, joint replacements, osteoporosis, constipation, indigestion, a headache or fatigue can cause people to resist whatever it is we are attempting to do with them. That is perfectly natural. Pain can interfere with both our ability to perform a task and our interest in doing so. Painful joints may make reaching down to tie our shoes a loathsome task; painful gums may cause us to avoid brushing our teeth.

As I've discussed at length in the companion book *Alzheimer's Basic Caregiving*, people with Alzheimer's disease often cannot express their pain directly, but may be "out of sorts" because of it. Watch for nonverbal signs of pain such as clenched jaws and hands, glazed eyes, frowning, and guarding behavior (protecting the painful area with an arm, for example).

Many people who are resistant to ADLs will become less so if they are regularly given an aspirin or other painkiller 15 minutes or so before initiating the uncomfortable task.

  Activities of daily living

If you suspect pain is at least a partial cause for resistance, talk with the person's doctor about giving an analgesic on a regular basis.

Uncomfortable in some other way

If we are tired, hungry or thirsty or need to use the bathroom, those needs may take precedence over any task. When I'm cold you'll remove my sweater at your peril, never mind trying to get me into a nightgown. The reverse of this, of course, is the resident who disrobes. Don't look for a sexual basis when the problem is more likely that she is too hot, her clothes are uncomfortable or she is sending a message that she needs to use the bathroom or go to bed for a nap.

Doesn't know who you are and feels exposed, vulnerable

Most people perceive being expected to take one's clothes off in front of strangers as an invasion of privacy. Even if you have helped him daily for a year, or lived with him for 50 years, especially in the late stages of Alzheimer's disease, you may be *perceived* as a stranger. And in the case of a female caregiver attempting to undress a male resident, you may be inadvertently sending a sexual message. Feeling exposed is a natural result of bathing and dressing, but there is much that can be done to protect people's modesty.

Failure to perceive a need for the procedure

- If I have Alzheimer's disease and I am comfortable in the clothes I am wearing, I may see no need to change from pajamas to street clothes (or vice versa) or to change clothes because I've spilled food on them or even because I smell bad (often unnoticed by aging people whose olfactory sense has diminished).

- You may think I need my beard shaved or my teeth brushed, but if I don't, it won't be easy to convince me, especially if I don't remember the steps (a fact I will never admit).

Reasons to resist care 9

You're not following the person's normal routine
People with Alzheimer's disease seem to be especially comforted by predictable routines.

- If she has always waited until after breakfast to groom herself or brush her teeth, trying to get her to do so before breakfast is likely to cause frustration and resistance.
- If she has always brushed her teeth and washed her face before changing into a nightgown for bed, you are going to upset her by trying to reverse that order.
- You can also upset someone by trying to get her up too early in the morning or trying to get her to retire too early in the evening.

On the other hand, if she's engaged in an activity she enjoys, she's not going to be interested in changing clothes or taking a bath even if it is part of a normal routine at that time.

The environment is upsetting or confusing
- If the room feels unfamiliar, is too hot or cold, or is poorly lit, people will often resist an activity. They need to feel both physically comfortable and emotionally safe. Remember that older adults need much more light to see clearly. The personal thermostats of older adults, especially people with AD, tend to go a bit haywire. A comfortable room temperature for them is likely to be considerably warmer than you think is necessary.
- Insofar as possible, eliminate unnecessary noise (blaring television, background music, vacuuming) that can interfere with a person's concentration for the task.
- Eliminate clutter, keeping in view only the props needed for that particular task or any specific distractions you plan to use to put the person at ease.
- An environment can also be confusing because it has too many people in it, including extra caregivers. (One

  Activities of daily living

exception can be group manicures which often have a pleasant beauty parlor atmosphere.)

- Institutional bathrooms are often downright scary. With rare exceptions, the resident bathrooms I've seen in institutions are not only undecorated, but drab (or sterile white) and completely unfamiliar-looking. This is especially problematic in long-term care settings where the bathtub or shower is in a separate room down the hall. Innovative bathtubs with a side-opening door may be wonderful for people with mobility problems, but they will still take some getting used to from the standpoint of the residents with dementia. And institutional showers often resemble car washes. If you wouldn't be comfortable bathing in that room, your residents won't be either.

Discomfort with the emotional atmosphere

- The person may feel rushed, pressure to perform, or undervalued by her caregiver.
- Environment can also have lingering effects. If a person was upset earlier by an argument between two people or a violent TV program, don't be surprised if the person continues to need reassurance that all is well, that she is safe and loved.

Miscellaneous reasons

Some (usually late-stage) people develop hypersensitive skin. With regard to dressing, that makes all but the softest cotton or flannel clothing feel prickly. They can't wear synthetics, and often need weighted vests or blankets to overcome their discomfort. A shower may feel like needles. (These people need to be rinsed instead with a washcloth firmly applied in downward strokes.) This is a more unusual problem, but should not be overlooked.

Communicating effectively

When attempting to gain a person's cooperation for any purpose, **never cause him to feel rushed** by your words, tone of voice or body language. When you enter his room to prepare him for a bath or help him dress, take a few minutes to reintroduce yourself if he has forgotten your name, and to chat about the weather or anything that is likely to put him at ease. Use a nurturing, reassuring approach. Assist only as needed. Be flexible. Look for ways to make the process pleasant.

Then keep these rules in mind:

Questions that can be answered "yes" or "no" should be asked only when you are willing to accept "no" for an answer. *Do you want to take a bath?* is not a question to ask when you are ready to bathe that person. Instead, try saying, *Your bath is ready now* or *It's bath time* and adding a reason the experience is likely to be pleasurable: *Here's your favorite lavender soap.*

Providing visual cues such as holding up a towel and soap or an outfit the person likes wearing helps orient the person with Alzheimer's disease to the task at hand. By lowering his confusion level, you are likely to heighten the chances for his cooperation.

Cajoling the person into bathing or giving logical explanations for why a bath is necessary **is likely to be futile.** People with dementia have their own logic based on their own perceptions of reality and often on their emotions. As I noted in the basic tenets and emphasized in the companion book, *Alzheimer's Basic Caregiving*, **you will never win an argument with someone who has AD**.

But if you forget these tenets and find yourself trying to reason with someone, excuse yourself, **walk away and try again a few minutes later,** or whenever the person is calm again. Alzheimer's expert consultant Mary Lucero offers this sage advice: *He can't resist if you don't insist.*

Once you get the person into the shower or start the process of dressing or brushing teeth, if the person is able to help herself and simply needs cueing, **give directions one step at a time. Use short sentences.** For example, *put your arm through this sleeve.* **Give her plenty of time to respond. Use props and gestures as back-up to your words.** For example, put the soap in her palm, hand her a toothbrush or give her a washcloth to scrub her face.

Speak in reassuring, positive tones. *MMMMmmm. Doesn't this lilac soap smell nice?* Then give her a chance to smell it; even if her olfactory sense is gone, chances are she'll have fond memories of the smell of lilacs. If she is able to handle all or most of the task on her own, **give her encouragement.** *You're doing great, Martha.* When she is successfully dressed, compliment her: *You look wonderful!*

If greater assistance from you is required, continue to **look for ways you can "do with" instead of "do for."**

- When bathing her, give her a chance to feel the water before she gets in to make sure it's a comfortable temperature. Ask her to hold the shampoo bottle. If you are using a handheld shower (as I recommend) as much as possible let her hold the shower nozzle and direct the spray herself, or try to give her some guidance by placing your hand gently over hers.
- When helping her put on her shoes, ask, *Would you please push your foot down into the heel?*
- When brushing her teeth, ask, *Would you mind holding the toothpaste?*

Always thank her for her help. When you must provide hands-on care, **explain each step of what you are doing.** In between explanations/directions, **speak conversationally** with the person. Ask how she's feeling today and if she has any particular aches or discomfort; pay attention to her answers! **Reposition her if necessary.**

Give her choices, but try to limit each choice to one of two things. *Would you like this rose-scented soap or the one that smells like lavender? Do you prefer to use a shower cap or go without? Do you want to use the pink towel or green one? Would you like to wear your blue dress or the one with pink flowers?* And always give the person time to respond before asking another question.

Look for ways to distract the person. Some people, especially as their dementia advances, need all their concentration to focus on the task at hand. Others who might be uncomfortable with the process can be put at ease by distracting them with conversation or a fiddle object.

- **Ask about daily events.** *Did you enjoy the performance by the 2nd graders who visited today? Aren't you glad spring weather has finally come?* Give her time to answer or to ask questions of her own.

- **Reminisce** with her based on what you already know about her. *Did you go to dances on Saturday nights? Did you have a favorite dancing partner? A favorite dance step?*

- **Sing. Tell jokes. Find reasons to laugh. Keep smiling.**

Activities of daily living

2—Dressing

*On the subject of dress almost no one,
for one reason or another, feels truly indifferent:
if their own clothes do not concern them,
somebody else's do.*
—Elizabeth Bowen

As the quote above suggests, we have a tendency to make harsh judgments on people – including ourselves – according to how they are dressed. Having a measure of vanity about our appearance generally signifies good mental health; when a person no longer cares about her appearance, it is often a sign of depression. We may have a favorite grunge outfit for washing the car, cleaning house or just watching TV, but most of us would be embarrassed to be seen in public wearing it. *Lookin' good!* is a compliment we all like to hear.

At the same time, we are embarrassed for others when we think their clothing reflects badly on them and sometimes embarrassed for ourselves to be seen with them. Prospective families looking for a long-term care setting (nursing home, assisted living, day care) for their loved one, are told to look at residents' clothing and appearance as one indication of the quality of care they are receiving. Yet conscientious caregivers know that judgments, particularly of people with Alzheimer's disease, need to be made with an understanding of the individual. If you see someone unusually dressed, it's better to be curious than quick to condemn. What does the clothing represent to that person?

Chapter 2: "Patterns of progression in Alzheimer's disease" in the companion book, *Alzheimer's Basic Caregiving – an ABC Guide* provides a fair amount of information on how interest in how one is dressed changes over time. This chapter focuses on how you can make the transitions work smoothly.

Ain't Misbehavin'

The perfect time to figuratively put yourself in the other person's shoes is when you are assisting with dressing.

Some people have what is called "visual agnosia" which is a loss of ability to identify what they see. In her book, *Speaking Our Minds*, author Lisa Snyder quotes a woman named Bea describing her difficulty in getting dressed:

One of the worst things I have to do is put on my pants in the morning. This morning I kept thinking there is something wrong because my pants just don't feel right. I had put them on wrong. I sometimes will have to put them on and take them off half a dozen times or more. I think I'm putting them on opposite of the way they are supposed to go on. It's so frustrating because I look at them and try to figure it out. I think I know the way to do it and I put them on and it's wrong again.

If you have been the caregiver of someone like Bea, you have probably thought, *How can it possibly take her an hour to get dressed?* But if you read her account, perhaps you can feel her disappointment when "doing her best" isn't enough. You may also be able to understand that once a person like Bea gets dressed, she is likely to want to stay in those same clothes as long as possible to avoid further frustration and confusion.

Learn individual past routines

As I noted throughout *Alzheimer's Basic Caregiving*, good care related to any ADL begins with knowing the person well.

- Where do dressing and undressing fall in the order of his preferred morning and nighttime routines for toileting, bathing or washing up? Does he have any other comforting rituals (For example, reading the morning paper in his pajamas, having a morning cup of coffee or bedtime snack, saying prayers)? What are the best (most alert, amenable) times for attempting morning dressing and evening undressing?

- Are there any special procedures or routines to keep in mind? (*Mother always puts her watch on her right wrist just after dressing . . . She puts on her glasses before she even gets out of bed, and needs them to see well enough to dress.*)

- What parts of the dressing and grooming process can she handle herself? How much prompting or assistance does she need?

- What are her favorite colors or favorite outfits? Are there any clothes or colors she dislikes or won't wear? (If so, get rid of them!)

- Are there any chronic illnesses or physical disabilities that may affect dressing? Is he taking any medications that might contribute to befuddlement, dizziness/balance or other conditions that interfere with dressing?

If you are a caregiver in a long-term care setting, don't hesitate to ask family members for any tips they can give you to make dressing an enjoyable part of the resident's day. Following are a few ideas.

Tips for dressing comfortably

You can help people to become more comfortable with the daily task of dressing (and most ADLs) when you:

A. Create an inviting environment

Assuming most grooming activities take place in the person's room where his furniture and familiar accessories are in place, the environment should already feel comfortable. In addition to the tips offered on page 10 are these:

- Keep only clothes that are appropriate to the current season (and a limited number of those) in the persons' closet or dresser drawers to **avoid confusion caused by too many choices.**

- **Lay the clothes out on a chair or bed in the order they are to be put on.** Recognize, however, that if you lay the clothes out the night before they are to be worn, some people may get up during the night and start dressing, cued by the clothes.

- **Be sure needed props are at hand,** such as a chair for steadying the person as he puts on his pants.

- Keep doors and, if appropriate, curtains closed to **ensure privacy.**

B. Use a reassuring, nurturing approach

- **Follow the person's individual preferences** and keep the routine as consistent as possible.

- **Always knock before entering the person's room, introduce yourself and let her know why you're there.** As Alzheimer's disease progresses, even family caregivers living at home with their loved ones may need to heed this advice.

- **Keep the person's comfort and safety uppermost in mind.** Be sure the clothes you are attempting to have the person wear fit well – loose enough to be comfortable (especially in waist and hips), not too long that they can be tripped on, and easy to get in and out of if necessary to prevent toileting accidents or simple frustration. **Make sure the clothes of people who are incontinent are easy to remove and care for.**

- **Pay attention to emotional comfort.** As described in Chapter 2 of *Alzheimer's Basic Caregiving*, in the early stages, people with Alzheimer's disease often want to dress to go out – make-up, jewelry, hose and purses for women; suits and ties, keys and wallet for men. Later on, they are less concerned with how they look to others or themselves and more concerned with what feels good to wear. (One potential signal of this change is their failure to recognize themselves in the mirror or their discomfort with this image.) This is not the time for stiff bras, binding girdles, control-top pantyhose, garters, tight belts, pinching earrings, or high-heeled shoes. Clothes that pull over and pull on or sweaters that button down the front or have oversized zipper pulls tend to make life easier for everyone. Some women will prefer to continue wearing dresses, but simply want looser-fitting ones. Others enjoy the comfort of sweat suits and tennis shoes. Respect people wherever they are in this progression and be accommodating.

- **As you simplify clothing in the later stages of Alzheimer's disease**, don't forget to **compensate for the change**. A woman who no longer wears a girdle and hosiery should not be left with bare legs, which can become cold easily, and which may make her feel half naked.

- **Assist only as needed**. In the early stages of Alzheimer's disease, the person may be able to maintain her independence if you simply organize her clothing, get rid of clutter and provide gentle reminders about changing clothes. In the middle stages, as noted previously, you may have to lay out the clothes in the order they are to be put on. Some people do well if you hand them each item in order. In the late stages, you will probably have to assist with every aspect of dressing.

- **Approach each task with a positive, matter-of-fact attitude and a belief in successful outcomes.** Expect her cooperation. She is more likely to accept your assistance if you ask for her help or suggest you can work on a task together than if you force her to admit she *needs* your help. (Not, *Here, let me do that for you*; rather, *Let's try this together*.)

- **Look for little things that might be uncomfortable**. Ladies used to be taught to smooth their skirts before sitting down, but may forget with Alzheimer's disease. Sitting on a bunched-up dress can be uncomfortable.

- **Respect the reasons why people change clothes frequently or add layers.** Some may be genuinely cold; some may have preferences overlooked by the caregiver. (For example, a man who likes long-sleeved shirts who is dressed in a short-sleeve shirt by a caregiver, may try to put another on over the first.) Some may be expressing another need. (For example, a woman who changes into her bathrobe in midday may be ready for a nap or not feeling well.) Some may simply be restless or indecisive and require another engaging activity. If a person in a long-term care setting has experienced her closet being mistaken for a department store by another resident, she may put on extra layers of clothes to protect them from being taken by the "shopper."

- Also **respect individual quirks**. A favorite purse, sweater, or hat may provide a sense of security and self-esteem that is of far greater value to the person than whether it looks attractive or "appropriate" to others.

- **Be flexible**. If you can only gain his cooperation long enough to change his shirt, save changing the pants until a little bit later. If he wants to sleep in the clothes he's worn during the day, and he's comfortable, what's the harm? Remember: *He can't resist if you don't insist.*

- **Look for ways to make the process pleasant.** Sing a silly song, reminisce about high button shoes, give the person a hug, tell her she looks smashing in that color, stop to watch the squirrels out the window. In the late stages, giving a person something to stroke or manipulate (furry fabric, a scarf, a beaded necklace) may enable you to proceed with dressing her easily. As noted on page 14, distractions can have a positive, calming effect

  Activities of daily living

and are needed for that purpose. On the other hand, some people need to focus all their attention on the particular task.

Tips for family shopping

- **If the person has a favorite outfit, try to purchase duplicates** of that outfit to provide opportunities for washing and changing the clothes.
- If the person has a favorite color or colors, **create a wardrobe that is color coordinated** so she can mix and match clothes at random.
- **Provide socks and shirts for men that will coordinate with any pair of pants** they choose.
- **Select colors with contrast** because they are easier to see, but avoid busy patterns which are distracting and may cause people with Alzheimer's disease to pick at their clothes.

Let's talk about feet

If it is well with your belly, chest and feet,
the wealth of kings can give you nothing more.
—Horace

When our feet hurt, we lose enthusiasm for every activity that requires their use, and may even be uncomfortable just sitting. As I've already noted, people with Alzheimer's disease often cannot express specific pain. Instead they show their discomfort through their behavior.

Many people with AD take their shoes off frequently. When this happens, first consider whether the shoes might be uncomfortable. Most people's feet are likely to swell during the day, especially if they spend much of their time sitting. Prop up the person's feet for part of the day. Also have a looser-fitting pair of shoes available. And, of course, examine the feet for in-grown toenails, bruises or other physical problems and treat as needed. Many people enjoy soaking their feet in warm water and Epsom salts. Foot rubs are a luxury to many who aren't overly ticklish. (Try it with peppermint lotion.)

Second, consider whether the person is removing his shoes because he is simply bored or restless and looking for something to do. Provide stimulating activities as needed.

Third, some people prefer bare feet because it helps give them a better sense of where their bodies are in space. They feel more grounded. (This is related to brain damage which interferes with their propriaception and vestibular sense.) Respect this need and educate families, staff and visitors, so they don't think you are being neglectful.

Bare feet are only a problem if the person is cold as a result, or if he has a tendency to stub his toes. Some people will willingly wear non-slip socks or more flexible footware.

Finally, some people will avoid wearing shoes because they don't know how to put them on (or simply can't bend any longer to do so) or don't feel safe in them. (This is not the time for high-heeled shoes for women.) Look for ways to simplify footwear. Tube socks don't have heels to line up. Velcro closures are easier to manage than laces. Slip-on shoes that don't slide off are usually easier for people to manage than tie shoes.

Activities of daily living

3 —Grooming

Ever since I put grease on my hair, everything slips my mind.
—*Author unknown, of course*

English is a complicated language, especially when you consider that we say our *nose runs* and our *feet smell.* Or that to *wind up a watch* is to start it, but to *wind up a speech* is to end it. One of my favorite ways to introduce the fact that it is easy to be misunderstood by people with Alzheimer's disease is to quote signs collected from foreign hotels written for their English-speaking customers:

- You are invited to take advantage of the chambermaid.
- Please leave your values at the front desk.
- Our wines leave you nothing to hope for.

It is usually when we believe we are making ourselves most clear that we are most likely to be misunderstood. People with Alzheimer's disease frequently misunderstand what is expected of them in essential grooming tasks. Here are some tips for making the process go more smoothly.

Nail care

- Soak both fingernails and toenails in warm water before cutting or clipping them. If a person has diabetes or particularly contentious toenails, take him to a podiatrist.

- Remember that a broken nail or ragged cuticle can be irritating and cause fidgeting, though the person with Alzheimer's disease is unlikely to be able to name the cause. Examine nails at least once daily, and file them regularly if the person cannot do so herself.

- Also clean beneath fingernails daily. Even bed-ridden people accumulate debris beneath their nails (probably from scratching dry skin).

- Some people with Alzheimer's disease seem to develop hypersensitivity in their nails; they will actually cry *ouch!* when their nails are cut, even when soaked first. Be gentle.

- On the other hand, many people, men and women, enjoy having a manicure, either for the attention or the pleasure of having hands held. Group manicures can add a chatty beauty parlor atmosphere, and you may find that those who are in earlier stages of AD enjoy providing nail care to those in later stages.

- Hand massages with lotion are great one-on-one or as an enjoyable group activity, with the benefits of moisturizing dry skin and stimulating circulation. However, be sensitive to arthritic hands.

- Use nail polish according to a woman's lifelong preferences. Some women love bright red nails, others are embarrassed by anything louder than clear polish.

Make-up

Be reasonable. In the early stages of AD, women will tend to want to continue with whatever make-up they have always worn. Others wear much less as they age and remain beautiful because their character shines through.

Husbands of women with Alzheimer's disease may want to take a few lessons from their wives while they are still able to say what they like and how to apply it – or by simple observation.

Eye make-up is usually the first thing to be abandoned because eye liner, shadow and mascara are particularly tricky to manage, especially if vision is poor and hands are unsteady. Caregivers are often at risk for poking the person in the eye with a mascara brush. Eye make-up is also often irritating to the eyes when they are rubbed, and it smudges easily. Many women, however, will continue to enjoy putting on lipstick and powdering their noses throughout their lives.

The bottom line here – as in so many aspects of care – is to honor what the person is comfortable with. Make-up is a lot like clothing. Maintaining a high standard is often more important to family members than to the person with AD. As Alzheimer's disease progresses, many people consider make-up an unnecessary bother. Then keep in mind Yoko Ono's advice: *Cosmetics are a boon to every woman, but a girl's best beauty aid is still a near-sighted man.*

Shaving

Retired bike racer Frankie Andreu had this advice about shaving legs: *The main thing is to not cut yourself and bleed to death in the tub.* That's good advice for everyone, but the bottom line is once again to honor individual preferences.

Most women with AD have little interest in shaving. As women age, the hair on their legs tends to thin out, and they sweat less (at least after the hot flashes of menopause). Indeed, because they are easily chilled, they may cover their legs with pants, tights, or stockings. Some women shave or pluck wayward facial hair, but the only reasons to continue shaving any part of women's bodies is their personal desire to do so, or to maintain their dignity in the face of others' insensitive comments. Then for safety, try an electric razor; painful measures such as waxing absolutely should not be attempted.

An unshaven man is much more visible than an unshaven woman because we tend to look at a person's face before her underarms or legs unless she's a contortionist. An unshaven man also tends to be more harshly judged by society. We are quick to label a man who can no longer shave himself (and who may object to others shaving him) as a "bum," and expect less gentlemanly behavior from him.

We then tend to feel justified in our judgment every time he is crabby, even when our persistence is what's causing the crabbiness. Here are the few tips I can offer, considering this is one grooming task that takes individual practice:

- Many men have always preferred the close shave they can achieve with a straight-edge razor or safety razor blade. Like women who have spent a lifetime peeling vegetables and can still handle a knife with aplomb, such men may be able to continue shaving themselves after other skills have diminished. Go with the person's preference as long as it's safe to do so, but don't hesitate to switch to an electric razor when necessary.

- Some men may be persuaded to puff out their cheeks and stretch their jaws from side to side to assist others in shaving them. Try to model the behavior you want from them.

- If you are a female professional caregiver, practice your shaving technique on your husband, brothers or grown sons, and ask their advice for how to make your residents more comfortable. Family caregivers can also ask for advice from other males in the family, including asking them to take over this task.

- Some women might find they can gain the man's cooperation by using the barber's trick of warm towels on the face. And actually having a barber shop shave in a barber shop chair is the best solution for some men, even if it can be done only once or twice a week.

- Author/expert and occupational therapist Carly Hellen has found that even when you have to perform the task for the person, you can help orient him to what's happening by putting a related item (such as a second shaver) in his hand.

- And some days the scruffy look unaccountably preferred by multiple movie stars may simply have to do.

26 **Activities of daily living**

Hair care

There are three ways a man can wear his hair:
parted, unparted and departed.
—Author Unknown

For several years after diagnosis, many women will still enjoy going to a beauty parlor for the full range of hair care, especially if that was a common lifetime experience. They may still have enough healthy vanity to want to have their hair permed or dyed or set in rollers. At some point, however, those procedures may become both uncomfortable and frightening. Then it is best to simplify hair styles either to a short, shapely cut or to long hair worn in a braid or French twist, based as much as possible on the person's preference.

One procedure that may continue to be enjoyed in a beauty-parlor-like setting is hair washing. Many people are uncomfortable having their hair washed in a shower, with water pouring down on their heads. Some people don't mind water pouring on their heads if it is not pouring on their bodies; washing one's hair at the kitchen sink was once a common procedure. Having our hair washed at a beauty parlor, however, with a scalp massage as an added bonus tends to be a lifelong luxury. Men tend to enjoy the barber shop version, too. (Even bald men enjoy a scalp massage.) But don't overdo it. Washing hair once or twice a week is adequate for most older people whose hair tends toward dryness anyway. Personally, I also prefer to avoid hair sprays and gels which build up residue on the hair and add another (sometimes upsetting) step.

A word of caution: Beauty parlors have chairs that tilt back and sink cutouts for necks. While not always perfectly comfortable, these help to minimize the stretching of the neck. However, tilting one's head backwards is risky for older adults, since it may interfere with the blood supply to the brain.

Technology has also brought us tear-free and rinse-free shampoos as well as a rinse-free shampoo cap that is heated in the microwave. Many of these products can be found at your local drugstore.

Many women (and men) enjoy having their hair brushed as a calming morning or bed-time ritual. When it is wet and freshly washed, however, be sure to use a large-tooth comb or a brush with widely-spaced, rubber-tipped bristles to gently remove tangles. For people with long hair, begin by combing out tangles an inch or two from the ends and slowly lengthen your strokes by working your way back toward the scalp.

Wigs fall into the same category as make-up; their usage should be determined by the person's comfort. Some older women have long been embarrassed by thinning hair, and wearing a wig is as important to them as wearing a blouse. However, at a certain point, that woman may find the wig itches or is too hot, and comfort becomes more important than vanity. Family members may have more trouble adjusting to the natural look than professional caregivers, but everyone deserves to be treated with dignity no matter how his or her outward appearance changes.

Eyeglasses

Most older adults wear glasses, but for a number of reasons many people with Alzheimer's disease are not wearing a prescription strength that is appropriate for them:

- Many older adults wear bifocals. The lower part of the lens is intended to enable them to read or do other close work without changing glasses as they look down. However, as Alzheimer's disease progresses, nearly everyone has a downward gaze, which means that many people are relying on their downward vision to assist them in knowing where to place their feet. Since the lower lens is meant to be used for a distance of about 12 – 18 inches, the person's feet inevitably look blurry through the lower lens. This can be disorienting and scary, increasing one's fear of falling.

- Other older adults use two or more pairs of glasses – one for reading and close work and one for watching TV or going to the movies, for example. As Alzheimer's disease progresses, they may lose the ability to choose the right pair of glasses for the right task.

- Between the ages of 50 and 80, it is not unusual for a person's eyeglass prescription to change multiple times, and not just because his vision is deteriorating with age. Most older adults are taking multiple medications, many of which can affect vision. If a medicine doesn't directly require a change in prescription, it may contribute to dizziness, balance problems, blurriness, (particularly early or late in the day), and dryness of the eyes. There have been many advances in eyeglass technology and ophthalmology, so that detecting disease and determining the curvature of a person's eyes can be done with minimal cooperation from the person. However, ultimately choosing the right prescription still comes down to choosing, *Is A clearer than B? Is B clearer than C?* Those are not answers a person with moderate to advanced Alzheimer's disease will be able to reliably give.

What does all this have to do with grooming? Essentially two things:

1. Many older people do not feel fully dressed without their glasses; it is up to us to help them to choose the right pair of glasses, and to watch for signs that a prescription may no longer be serving their

needs. In residential care settings, this means it is essential to label glasses with the person's name and to keep a description of the glasses in that person's record.

2. If a person repeatedly removes her glasses or shows signs of agitation or discomfort wearing them, you can be quite sure the glasses are dirty, don't belong to her (a common problem in residential care settings) or are of a prescription strength that no longer works for her. Pay attention and make the necessary changes. Sometimes wearing no glasses is better than wearing an inappropriate prescription.

Many older adults also have dry eyes and would benefit from having eyedrops added to their everyday grooming routines.

Finishing touches

Knowing what pleases an individual also extends to accessories. Here are a few things to keep in mind:

- Jewelry: Many people do not feel fully dressed without a watch, even if they can no longer tell time, don't need to, or the watch doesn't work. Women often feel naked without rings on their fingers. If valuable rings are a concern, especially in residential care settings, try substituting costume jewelry. Many women also like to complete their outfits with pins, earrings, necklaces or bracelets.

- Others may want to add a scarf or hat. The latter can also keep both men and women's heads warm when hair is thin.

As long as any of these things increase people's pleasure in daily grooming, indulge their vanity.

- Honor the person's sense of self. Many women, at least through the moderate stage of AD, like to carry purses.

  Activities of daily living

Men tend to like to complete their outfits with keys, wallets and a bit of change, even if they have no use for any of those things on a given day. These items are strongly tied to people's identities, and may take on added significance as a person faces other losses. For example, a woman may carry a house key (representing "home"), photos (her family and friends), lipstick (her beauty parlor), a band-aid or pills (her medicine cabinet/first aid kit), some money (financial security), and gum (emergency food).

Never underestimate the importance of these finishing touch items in helping a person navigate the day confidently.

4—Oral Hygiene

No matter how grouchy you're feeling,
You'll find the smile more or less healing.
It grows in a wreath
All around the front teeth -
Thus preserving the face from congealing.
~Anthony Euwer

Talk to any infection control nurse, and she will tell you that the number one rule for protecting ourselves from others' germs is to wash our hands often. This includes not only scrubbing with soap and running water (paying attention to nails and cuticles), but also turning off faucets and opening the door with clean paper towels as one leaves a public bathroom.

Two other things are also important for infection control: the first is to relax. Stress lessens our ability to fight off disease by compromising our immune system. That, of course, is easier said than done. One thing that increases stress for care receivers is being asked to do something they don't want to do or don't understand how to do. One thing that increases stress for caregivers is trying to get their care receivers to do those things.

One task people with Alzheimer's disease often resist is oral hygiene, and it is also one task caregivers often don't push. However, your mouth is not only the window to what is going on in the rest of your body, but the doorway for many infections. That makes good oral hygiene the third most important weapon against infection. Ask any dentist.

Smiling for the health of it

There is no disputing that smiles can contribute to our well being and our ability to connect with one another, but less attention has been paid to the connection between our mouths and our overall health.

Articles provided by MayoClinic.com, Colgate (www. colgate.com) and the Wisconsin Dental Association (www. wda.org) indicate that:

- There is a strong correlation between poor oral hygiene and an increased risk of heart attack, stroke, poorly controlled diabetes and complications related to rheumatoid arthritis, among other conditions.
- Proper oral hygiene is also protective in maintaining the body's natural immune system.
- When our teeth and gums are in good condition, we are more likely to enjoy eating, and therefore eat well. Healthy eating promotes healthy teeth.

In other words, brushing your teeth is not just good for your smile, but for your whole body.

Older adults who fail to maintain good oral hygiene habits are at increased risk for ill health because:

1. Cavities and decay on the root surfaces of teeth are more common in older adults. (Dentists recommend a fluoride toothpaste.)
2. Many older adults have increased tooth sensitivity which may make them less inclined to brush. (This increased sensitivity may be an indication of a more serious problem such as a cavity or cracked tooth.)
3. Gum recession and gum diseases tend to increase with age. Receding gums have the effect of making teeth more susceptible to decay and more difficult to brush adequately.
4. Dry mouth, technically called xerostomia, is a common condition in older adults. According to Thomas J. Hughes, DDS, president of the Wisconsin Dental Association, "Saliva is the mouth's self-

cleansing mechanism. It helps remove food debris and plaque from tooth surfaces." When saliva decreases, the risk for cavities and oral diseases increases. Dry mouth can also affect a person's speech, taste sensation and ability to swallow. People with dry mouth usually complain of a sore or burning sensation on the tongue, dry, cracked lips and at the corners of the mouth, and they are often thirsty. This condition is frequently related to a broad range of diseases, radiation therapy and many common medications, such as decongestants, diuretics, antihypertensives, antidepressants, and antihistamines.

Bacteria from our mouths don't normally enter our bloodstream, but invasive dental treatments – sometimes even just routine brushing and flossing if we have gum disease – can provide a port of entry. Medications that reduce saliva flow and antibiotics that disrupt the normal balance of bacteria in our mouths can also result in compromised defenses that allow these bacteria into our bloodstream. When our immune systems are healthy, oral bacteria in our blood stream don't usually cause problems, but when our immune system is weakened, oral bacteria in our blood stream may cause us to develop a serious infection in another part of our body.

Brushing teeth

People should brush their teeth a minimum of twice a day, and ideally after each meal as well as upon rising and before bed. People in the early stages of AD may simply need to be reminded to do so, but as their brain deteriorates, chances are they will need increasing verbal and even physical guidance.

Begin by verbally breaking the task into simple steps. Wait until each step is completed before giving the next direction. *Take the cap off the toothpaste . . . Pick up the toothbrush . . . Squeeze some toothpaste on the brush . . . Now put the brush in your mouth . . .* Be patient in waiting for each step to be completed. If you have to repeat an instruction, use the same words. It may take awhile for the person to absorb your directions, so don't automatically assume you weren't heard or understood if the person takes no immediate action.

Some caregivers find that beginning the process for the person enables him to continue from there — for example, handing him a toothbrush with toothpaste already on it.

Eventually you may actually have to guide the person's hand or take over the task of brushing and flossing the person's teeth. No caregiver should brush or floss the teeth of someone with Alzheimer's disease until she has experienced having her own teeth brushed and flossed by another person. I assure you this is a jaw-dropping lesson in sensitivity. Most of us do not realize how invasive it can feel. Our discomfort is compounded if we have a sensitive tooth or sore gums. Face the person, position yourself at eye level, move slowly and gently (quick movements increase fear) and explain what you're doing while you're doing it.

Here are a few more tips:

- As with shaving, author and occupational therapist Carly Hellen has found that if you must brush the person's teeth, you can often help orient him to the task by giving him a duplicate prop to hold – in this case a second toothbrush.

- Some people need to expend all their concentration on the task. Others can be put at ease if you offer some distraction. Sing a toothpaste jingle, talk about favorite toothpaste flavors, talk about how animals clean their teeth (dogs on bones).

  Activities of daily living

- Though it may sound silly, some people can follow directions more easily if you sing them. It not only sets the directions into a rhythm (helping to make them more memorable) but also helps to create a beat for the action desired. You don't even have to have a good voice, as I can attest. If any readers remember the old Ipana toothpaste commercials from the 1950s in which the beaver sang, *Brusha, brusha, brusha*, you'll know what I mean.

- Try to use the person's favorite style of toothbrush (soft bristles are essential) and favorite brand of toothpaste to breed familiarity. If a person is living in the past, you might revert to his childhood form of toothpaste, which may have been a powder, or baking soda.

- On the other hand, don't be afraid to try something new. A person who has become resistive to brushing may be persuaded to take up a toothbrush if you use a bubble-gum-flavored or other sweet toothpaste. And some people react well to electric toothbrushes, even if it's a new experience. (Indeed, since electric toothbrushes tend to do a much better job of cleaning, I am a strong proponent of helping people to adjust to this method.) Experiment. Give the person at least several weeks to adjust.

- Give gums the same attention as teeth. Massage gums to dislodge plaque and food debris.

- For proper hygiene, remember to replace toothbrushes every 60 days.

Late stage brushing tips

There's a wise saying, *When things go wrong, don't go with them.* As Alzheimer's disease progresses, brushing teeth may become a major anxiety-producer for both you and the person you're caring for. Look for other ways to cleanse the mouth.

- Some people can handle swishing and spitting longer than brushing. Use mouthwashes for them. Avoid alcohol-based brands for people with dry mouth.

- Don't use mouthwash if a person tends to swallow it. Switch to following meals with a drink of water. This tends to remove bits of food in the mouth and aids hydration.

- Consider toothpicks. Many people – men especially – have had a lifelong habit of removing food particles with a toothpick after meals. This is a good practice to maintain when flossing becomes more difficult. Get a toothpick dispenser and encourage this practice. Be sure to throw out the used toothpicks so they don't become a health or safety hazard.

- If swallowing gum or proper disposal is not a problem, sugarless chewing gum can also be an imperfect but feasible means of freshening breath and cleaning teeth.

- If even soft bristles are rejected by the person, try using a small, damp washcloth or a gauze pad to gently wipe the person's teeth.

- Use the disposable flavored sponges that are used for swabbing the mouths of hospital patients who are not allowed to eat or drink for a period of time. The sponges are much gentler than brushes and the flavor is often appealing. However, lemon-flavored swabs are not recommended for people with dry mouth.

Denture care

Most people with dentures take them out at night for a good soak-cleansing, but many do not brush them or remove them after every meal, unless food particles caught between the dentures and gums have made them uncomfortable. If the person with dentures does not want to cleanse them after meals, he should at least be encouraged to rinse his mouth with water or mouthwash after each meal to get rid of food particles. Following is the basic procedure for night-cleansing:

1. Have the person rinse with water to loosen food particles and the dentures before removal.

2. If the person needs your assistance in removing the dentures, be sure to wash your hands with a disinfectant soap before reaching into his mouth. (Residential care settings require the use of rubber gloves as well since this involves contact with saliva, a body fluid.) Break the suction on the top teeth by pulling from the side and from the bottom teeth by putting your thumb and forefinger on either side of the front teeth and lifting. As this is an invasive procedure, be sure to talk to the person to explain what you're doing and put him at ease.

3. Using toothpaste, brush dentures thoroughly and rinse them. Place them in a cup of water and add a cleansing tablet. Let them soak until morning.

In the morning, rinse the dentures before putting them back in the person's mouth. Using warm (not hot) water will heat them close to body temperature, which may make them feel less foreign or shocking. Most people have a preference for putting either tops or bottoms in first – usually tops. Honor that preference.

A few other tips:

- As Alzheimer's disease progresses, body changes (including weight loss or gain) may alter the fit of dentures, making them uncomfortable and inefficient. A dentist can create a better-fitting set. Poor fitting dentures may also collect food particles between the teeth and gums, adding to their discomfort. Since people with Alzheimer's disease lose their ability to verbalize their pain as their brain deterioration increases, you will need to recognize it in other ways, such as grimacing while eating or refusing to eat. Some people who are uncomfortable are just plain cranky. One clear way you will know it's time for an adjustment is when the dentures slip around in a person's mouth or when they are repeatedly removed by the person.

- Labeling dentures with a person's name is essential. It is not unusual for a person with Alzheimer's disease to remove her dentures and leave them in odd places and, in residential care settings, not unusual for them to be picked up by another resident and "shared." Permanent labels can be incorporated when the dentures are made and dentures can also be engraved with their owners' name at a later date, such as when a person enters an assisted living community.

- When something is useless or objectionable, we discard it. Therefore, always check wastebaskets before emptying and toilets before flushing for discarded dentures (also hearing aids, glasses, clip on earrings, etc.)

- Some people are able to wear their dentures until they die, but others seem to prefer life without them fairly early on. Respect the person's preference. Ill-fitting dentures may be able to be replaced by better-fitting ones. However, let us not judge others according to the physical alteration caused by a toothless grin. Many people are able to speak and eat and go about their daily lives remarkably well without their teeth. Celebrate that strength.

Going to the dentist

There is really only one tenet: Choose carefully. If the person with AD has had a long relationship with a particular dentist, a little cueing of the dentist on how to handle her now that she has developed Alzheimer's disease may suffice. Other people find it works better to choose a dentist who has experience in working with the elderly and maybe even specializes in Alzheimer's disease care. Some residential care homes provide an in-house dental office and bring in a dentist on a regular basis to simplify the process and shorten the time involved.

If you must go out to a dental office:

- Schedule the appointment for a time when the person is likely to be alert, and preferably the first patient of the day or the first patient after lunch, to avoid waiting room time.

- Many people are terrified of the dentist. Some people have had truly painful experiences in dental offices, especially if they developed cavities before the days of high speed drills and other more recent innovations. Others are simply uncomfortable with the array of devices dentists manage to cram into their mouths. (Gary Larsen created a Far Side cartoon of a dentist's office with the caption, *Let's just see if we can get this tennis ball in, too.*) For people who are fearful of the dentist, a mild tranquilizer before the appointment may be in order.

- Look for ways to make the visit pleasant or more familiar. As a family caregiver, you may be able to help the person into the dental chair and even stay close by holding her hand or arm, if that's logistically possible. Some people are comforted by favorite music played through ear phones. Others can be bribed by the promise of a treat after the appointment.

- Ask for the dentist's advice. One man who was unable to get his wife to brush her teeth at all found a dentist who would clean them in his office quarterly, and this sufficed. Dentists can also prescribe mouthwashes to help prevent puffy and bleeding gums that can lead to gingivitis and other problems. (One brand name is Peridex, but my dentist simply supplied a formula for combining baking soda and hydrogen peroxide.) Dentists can also recommend special brushes, picks, and cleansers.

5 —Continence Care

Could the term "no fly zone" also be applied
to a women's bathroom?
—Ross Baker

The topic of this chapter is continence care, or what is generally referred to by staff in residential care settings as "toileting," a subject and a word most of us prefer to avoid for its graphic unpleasantness.

Our word choices are limited by the English language, but the subject matter is unavoidable when we talk about Alzheimer's disease. The reality is that brain deterioration eventually causes everyone with AD to become incontinent of bowel and bladder. However, many people with AD, both at home and in long-term care settings, become prematurely incontinent because they are not toileted regularly or their toileting needs go unrecognized. As a result of too many "accidents," they are put in Depends or a related product. Whatever the reasons for toileting difficulties, many family members who have valiantly cared for their loved ones at home for years become extremely uncomfortable when they must change a spouse's or parent's incontinence product. Indeed, incontinence is one of the top three reasons families choose to place their loved ones with Alzheimer's disease in a long-term care residence.

Nevertheless, urinating and defecating are as natural as breathing, and as vital to our health. To make a bad pun, we cannot afford to be anal about this topic.

Ain't Misbehavin'

I know of no long-term care setting which has not had to deal with residents' creative locations for relieving themselves. Dresser drawers, waste baskets and potted palms seem to be particular favorites. But notice I called these choices "creative" rather than "inappropriate." It's important to recognize that when residents are not using a toilet, they are doing the best they can with a damaged brain. There is always a logical reason for their choices.

One of the most common reasons for using a non-toilet for toileting purposes is an inability to find the bathroom. Bathrooms should be well-marked. Many long-term care settings have designed resident rooms so that the bathroom – and specifically the toilet – is visible from the person's bed to make it easy to relieve night-time urges. Since it is not always possible to leave public restroom doors open – and people may still miss them while walking down the hallway if they have diminished peripheral vision – creative signage has been tried with varied success. People with Alzheimer's disease can usually read until quite late into the disease process, although not necessarily with comprehension. Nevertheless, the words "restroom" and "toilet" can be recognized by many for a long time and those words on the door eliminate the frustration of a woman who can only find the men's room and vice versa. A graphic of a toilet on the door will work for some people with Alzheimer's disease, but symbols lose their meaning earlier than words for others. Residential care designers have sometimes found it helpful to put a brightly colored awning over the bathroom door so that it is visible from a distance. However, as their brain damage progresses, people with Alzheimer's disease tend to have a downward gaze. Eye level signage is what is generally required by federal ADA (Americans with Disabilities Act) regulations, but it is probably wise to have a backup landmark. One idea is to hang a brightly colored quilt next to each public restroom that is visible from both near and far to people with AD.

Another common reason people with AD relieve themselves in unusual places or have accidents is that they recog-

  Activities of daily living

nize the need too late. Sometimes this is related to apraxia, the inability to initiate and carry out previously learned complex tasks. They may no longer know how to undress themselves or they have trouble sequencing actions. Others may know what to do, but cannot follow through with the motor movements required. (For example, arthritis may prevent a person from certain actions or poor vision may compromise a man's aim.) Sometimes it simply takes them awhile to tune into their bodily needs, in the same way that you may have to call a person by name three times before he tunes in to your voice. They may be unaware that their bladder is full until it is just about to empty and they do not make it to the bathroom in time. This is especially true at night, which is why a bedside commode helps some people.

It must also be said that what is an "unusual" spot to void for some, may not be for others. If you are located in a farming community, or if the person in question has led a predominantly outdoor life, especially in youth or as a young adult, urinating behind the nearest tree may seem far more natural than seeking indoor plumbing.

Many toileting accidents, however, have a physiological cause. As people age, they may suffer a decrease in bladder muscle tone or a weakening of sphincter muscles. Women may have a prolapsed uterus or atrophic vaginitis due to lack of estrogen. Men may have a variety of prostate problems. Stress incontinence – leakage caused by laughing, coughing or sneezing – is also common in older adults, with or without Alzheimer's disease.

More serious (but usually curable) physiological causes are illnesses and infections. Remember that as Alzheimer's disease progresses, people lose their "self-reporting" abilities. They may seem listless, but they cannot tell you that they are having a burning sensation when they urinate or that they feel pressure to urinate, but can't. Bladder and urinary tract infections are extremely common and often go undetected far too long.

However, incontinence of urine may actually be caused by constipation. A person who is constipated may lose bladder control due to the pinching off of the urinary outlet. As a safeguard to keep the bladder from bursting, the body releases urine in trickles and spurts. Obviously, the impaction should be treated.

It can be dangerous to a person's health to fail to recognize constipation, but on the other hand, both caregivers and care receivers can become unnecessarily anxious about the lack of a daily BM. A soft, formed stool should be passed without strain at least three times a week, but not everyone has a bowel movement daily. Using laxatives to increase the frequency of bowel movements is a dangerous practice. It can lead to the disappearance of nerve cells, making it impossible to defecate without chemical stimulation. A high-fiber diet, plenty of liquids and regular exercise are the chief factors in establishing a normal pattern of bowel movements.

Other medical conditions – out of control diabetes or heart failure, for example –can also cause incontinence and go undetected. If a person comes to associate the bathroom with discomfort, she is likely to avoid going there, and the incontinence problem can quickly escalate.

In addition, medications used to treat other problems often have an effect on bladder and bowels. Tranquilizers, hypnotics and sedatives affect urine control. Excedrin and aspirin contain caffeine, a bladder irritant. Some high blood pressure medicines also irritate the bladder. Anti-Parkinsonian medications and antihistamines can cause urinary retention which may lead to infection or dribbling of urine. Some medications, including certain antibiotics, cause diarrhea; others cause constipation. Some drugs

Activities of daily living

increase befuddlement and "fuzzy thinking" which interfere with a person's ability to toilet herself independently. For any suspected physiological problem, whether it is caused by disease or drugs, consult a physician.

Finally, don't underestimate the role of psychological factors. A person who is frustrated, angry or depressed by his AD may develop bladder or bowel problems. Many of us have suffered from diarrhea when under extreme stress, for instance. Feeling rushed or pressured or sensing a caregiver's impatience or irritation can also affect toileting independence. Anxiety over the need to have a bowel movement, as noted earlier, can result in psychological stress.

Whenever you are having a problem with a person with Alzheimer's disease, remember that it's easier to change your habits than his. Ask, *What could I be doing differently?*

Use words that the resident understands

If you are caring for a family member, you know him well and know his toileting habits and terms. When placing him in a long-term care setting, be sure to share this information with staff. Effective communication is the first step toward maintaining continence. Respect privacy by being unobtrusive when assisting someone to the bathroom, but make your intent clear. Most people understand the simple phrase, *It's time to use the bathroom.*

Others may require you to be more delicate. Some women, are quite prim and prefer terms like "commode" and "powder room." Other people may more clearly understand slang terms such as "can," "john," "loo," "head," or the military term, "latrine." Go with what works, both for the location and the function, and don't waste time being offended by terms you consider crude, or make fun of people whose terminology you find amusing.

My experience leads me to believe that nurses and sailors are blasé about all language having to do with body parts and functions. Most others blush easily. Using the right words with the right person is important.

Avoid dehydration

If you are a family caregiver who has had your sleep interrupted for the second time during the night for the third night in a row by a loved one who has wet the bed, or if a male resident is upsetting female residents by urinating in the geraniums, it is tempting to withhold liquids. **Never treat incontinence by withholding adequate liquids in that person's diet.** Limiting the intake of liquids makes the urine more concentrated, resulting in irritation to the bladder, which can lead to infections. Inadequate liquid intake also contributes to constipation, increased falls, and added confusion.

First evaluate what's normal for this person. Recognize that frequency of urination increases with age, particularly at night. Night-time wandering of people with Alzheimer's disease is often triggered by the need to use the bathroom. People with AD put out as much urine at night as during the day, and this tends to become more challenging as the disease progresses. You may also find that urination increases in cold weather.

If the episodes of incontinence represent a change in pattern, particularly a sudden one, check with a physician, preferably a urologist, for a possible medical reason.

Then evaluate diet. Limit the intake of coffee, tea, colas and other products with caffeine which may irritate the bladder or cause frequent urination. (Caffeine is a diuretic.) Substitute water and juice (but recognize that citrus juice is also a bladder irritant for some people) or decaffeinated coffee and herbal teas. For those who are not lactose intolerant, milk is also a good choice. You can also hydrate a person with water-rich solids such as Jell-o, popsicles, ice cream and some of the juicier fruits.

To prevent dehydration (a topic discussed more thoroughly in Chapter 7), everyone needs a minimum of six glasses of liquid per day (1-1/2 quarts). Whenever a person indicates he is thirsty, always provide something to drink. Over time people with Alzheimer's disease lose their ability to ask for something to drink, to provide it for themselves or even to recognize it when it is placed in front of them. It's up to you to make sure their intake is adequate.

If constipation is a concern, add fresh or dried fruits (especially apricots, pears, grapes, raisins, dates, and prunes) and raw vegetables, wheat germ, bran and whole wheat flour to the person's diet. If diarrhea is a problem, cheese and bananas are usually good at binding the bowels.

Keep to a schedule

People with Alzheimer's disease tend to do well when following a predictable routine. Use this to your advantage, and **set up a regular toileting schedule with the person**. This is probably the single most important factor in maintaining continence. In the beginning, take the person to the bathroom (or encourage him to go if he doesn't require assistance) when he gets up in the morning, after breakfast, and after that, every two hours throughout the day (and the night, if necessary). You will soon be able to tell if he needs to use the bathroom more often or less. But once you have determined the comfortable intervals between toileting, stick to that schedule.

Additional tips

Beyond that, here are some other tips:

A. Create a clean and inviting environment.

- The advantage of home bathrooms is that they look familiar and often cozy. In long-term care settings, try to achieve that same coziness.

- Use multiple nightlights for nighttime way-finding. Many falls among the elderly occur after they have turned out the bathroom light and are attempting to return to bed before their eyes have adjusted to the change.

- Within each bathroom, make the toilet as visible as possible. A white toilet against a white wall and white tile floor is difficult for people with deteriorating vision to see clearly. Some people have found success using a strongly colored toilet seat or painting the rim of the toilet basin deep blue or green, thus creating a bull's eye for men to aim for. Others have found that painting the walls around the toilet in a strongly contrasting color helps the toilet to stand out better in the person's eyes.

- Use bathroom aids like a raised toilet seat and grab bars. (This is essential for people who have broken a hip or have hip pain.) A padded seat is conducive for encouraging some people to sit awhile. A basket of magazines may add to an unhurried atmosphere and reinforce old patterns, especially in men.

B. Use a reassuring approach.

- Allow people as much privacy as possible.

- If you must help with all aspects of toileting, do so in a matter-of-fact manner, without making a big deal of it.

- Be alert to cues that a person may need to use the restroom. Watch for fidgeting, pulling at clothes, anxious wandering, etc.
- NEVER scold or belittle a person who soils his clothing or voids/defecates in an inappropriate place. He is doing the best he can with a damaged brain and is likely to feel embarrassed or humiliated already. Simply say, *Don't worry. I'll help you get cleaned up.*
- If you are taking a resident to the bathroom on a regular basis, do so unobtrusively, especially when the resident is involved in a group activity. NEVER announce to everyone present, *Mrs. Jones, it's time for you to go to the bathroom.* Consider offering an invitation: *Mrs. Jones, I'd love it if you would come for a little walk with me.*
- As confusion worsens, assist as needed, but to help maintain independence, give instructions one step at a time: *Pull down your pants . . . Sit down . . . You can go now . . . Now wipe yourself.*
- When you are helping someone to the bathroom at night, reduce his fear and confusion by identifying yourself and explaining what you are doing.
- Sometimes getting the person to give you a bear hug while you pull down his pants and lower him to the toilet seat works effectively. (Note that men may find urinating while seated is easier than their lifelong pattern, now that they are less steady on their feet and with their aim.)

C. Miscellaneous tips and techniques
- Simplify clothing. If a person can't manage a belt and zipper, try pants with an elasticized waist. Some women, on the other hand, may find it easier to pull up a skirt than pull down pants.

- If someone is having trouble getting started voiding, use the old "run the faucet" trick to stimulate reflexes.

- For a person who does not want to stay sitting long enough to void or defecate, giving the person something to concentrate on or fiddle with can help. Besides the old standby of magazines, you might try jewelry, a manipulative gadget, knotted socks or an appealing scarf or other piece of fabric.

Incontinence tips

- Most people are uncomfortable with the term "diapers" when used in reference to an adult. Look for a term that is acceptable to the person. Some people go with the brand name (Depends or Attends), others talk of "pads" or "new underwear." You may have other ideas.

- Some people are aware the minute they wet or soil their incontinent product (or their clothes, if incontinence is only occasional), and may fidget or try to remove the offending clothes/product. Others are oblivious to being soiled, but may disturb others by the odor they give off. To prevent rashes, chafing and infections, change incontinent products as often as you had previously taken that person to the bathroom when he was continent, or sooner if you realize his clothes/products are soiled.

- If the person is aware of being wet or soiled, acknowledge his feelings. *You must be uncomfortable. Let's make you feel better.*

- Skin care of the incontinent person is vital. After each episode of incontinence, the skin should be washed with soap and water, dried with a towel and swabbed with protective skin products. Alcohol-free and fragrance-free moisturizing lotions help prevent cracking of dry skin. Protective ointments, such as A&D also help.

(Vaseline should be avoided since it does not allow the skin to breathe.)

Finally, remember as in all things, experiment to find what works for the person at this point in time. **The right angle for tackling a problem is the "try-angle."**

6—Bathing

Half of the secret of resistance to disease is cleanliness;
the other half is dirtiness.
—Anonymous

If you are a home caregiver, the bathroom is likely a familiar place, and often a cheery one – Americans seem to have a penchant for adding humorous touches to their bathrooms. One of my favorites is a Florida friend who uses a pink flamingo's beak as a toilet paper holder. As noted in Chapter 1, most institutional settings could enhance their bathroom environments by adding more whimsical touches – or at least pretty towels, scrubbable wallpaper and a few plants.

But a cozy environment does not guarantee bathing success. Virtually all of the reasons for resisting other activities of daily living also apply to bathing. And there are others:

- **Fear of falling,** perhaps based on past experience in a slippery tub or shower.
- **Fear of the water.** Although no one seems quite sure why, this is common among people with AD.
- **Uncomfortable being naked** in front of others the person perceives as strangers, even if they are long-time caregivers or family members. Sometimes family members – especially adult children of the opposite sex – contribute to this discomfort because they are uncomfortable bathing their parent and the person with AD picks up readily on those non-verbal cues. (Over time, **consistency in caregivers helps enormously.**)
- **Unwillingness to take off a favorite piece of clothing** or item which provides security. (You *can* bathe him with his baseball cap and glasses on.)

A word to families

One of the reasons family members sometimes have difficulty bathing a parent or spouse is the caregiver's tendency toward standoffs. The family caregiver is ready to give a bath, but the care receiver is fearful of the process or simply tired and refuses. The family member says, *Aw, come on. It's been three days and you smell bad.* That gives the care receiver something new to argue about, and he angrily retorts, *I do not!* The battle has begun.

A better approach, at least in the earlier stages when the person may have lost some interest in personal hygiene but can still plan an action and follow through is to agree on a compromise. You will only ask him to bath three or four times a week and will draw up a calendar with "Xs" to mark the bath days. In exchange for his agreement not to argue, you agree not to nag.

Following are other ideas.

Putting the person at ease

Because bathing is such an intimate activity, as well as one which involves a number of steps perceived as complex for the person with AD, finding ways to help the person relax is particularly important. The key is to know the individual and remain flexible in meeting his special needs. As already noted, a person who doesn't want to remove a favorite hat or glasses can be bathed with them on. A woman who is excessively modest can be soaped and rinsed while being covered with towels (through or under them) or, if she prefers, by keeping her underwear on like a bathing suit and spraying soap and water through the extra layer. (She will be more willing to change the underwear once it is wet.)

Distraction is another way to help a person relax. Singing in the shower where echoes enhance any voice can be especially satisfying. Alzheimer's consultant Mary

Lucero says a study found that a rubber ducky is the most universally understood symbol of bath time, even for people who never bathed with one. Having learned that, I have begun a collection of rubber duckies which come in an incredible range of "uniforms," such as: king and queen, devil, Hawaiian (with lei), birthday (with cake or present in wings), bride and groom, pirate, sailor, snorkeler, celebrities (Mae West and many more). They also come with dozens of hats and in nearly every color. (One source: ....) Keep a few on hand. The number of rubber squeeze objects and balls is enormous. Some people may be offended by being given a rubber ducky to hold, but most will be amused, especially if given an odd variation. (*Isn't it amazing what people conceive of making?*) Or use the toy to reminisce about bath and pool amusements. I also favor red squeezable rubber hearts (which I hand to the person with the words, *Here's a little symbol of my love for you to hold*), yellow smiley face balls and food that can get wet. (Grapes and strawberries are two possibilities, but be mindful of residents prone to choking.)

A few basic considerations

As always, know the person well. **Try to bathe him:**

- **At the time of day or evening when he was used to bathing.** For instance, men who were laborers may have showered after work, but before dinner. Others were accustomed to taking a shower each morning before breakfast and still others bathed only on Saturday nights.

- **When he is most alert.** We hope these times coincide, but if they don't, experiment to see which works best. In the early stages of AD, old routines may be key. Later, as people have more difficulty remembering the multiple steps involved in bathing, simply concentrating can be exhausting, and choosing the "most alert" time may be more important.

Personal preferences go beyond time and frequency of bathing. Does the person prefer quick showers or languid bubble baths? Washing her hair in the shower or the kitchen sink? Rinsing with a wash cloth or shower spray?

Some **people are used to following a detailed sequence of events**, e.g., *run the water, use the toilet, get undressed, get into the tub, wash herself from top down, get out of the tub and dry off, put on pajamas (tops first), have a snack of milk and graham crackers, brush her teeth, get into bed.* Know and honor as far as possible those preferred sequences. The comfort of set routines is based on their sequence, not precise timing.

Also **be aware of special issues.** Is he a holocaust survivor? If so, do not use the word "shower" and be especially careful to make the bathing room home-like.

Vision deficits can also create problems. Some people are more comfortable when the bath water is colored with a bath oil, gel or salts; clear water is hard to see and adds to confusion. (However, bath oils can leave a slippery residue in the tub.) Contrasting colors between walls and tub or shower also increase visibility.

Many older people have **hearing impairments.** Running water is a noise distraction that can interfere with normal conversation. In addition, bathrooms often echo, and while this is fun when you're singing, it can cause confusion when you're trying to give someone directions. Room decorations, towels and rugs can help diffuse reverberating sounds.

You can sometimes prevent toileting "accidents" in the shower if you run the bath water before the person enters the room, and give her a chance to use the toilet just before she takes a bath (or run the water while she's sitting *on* the toilet). The device which was indispensable in caring for my mother during the late stage of her AD was a PVC shower chair with a mesh back (for soaping and spraying through) and a commode seat. When the removable pan was in place, it caught her bowel movements which bathing seemed to stimulate, (often the case in people who are non-ambulatory) and when it was removed, it was easy to clean her perineal area. The four-wheeled chair allowed her to remain safely seated before, after, and during bathing.

For those who have a **fear of falling** or are at risk to fall, look into the wide range of bath and shower safety aids, including the PVC chair just mentioned. Use grab bars and rubber safety strips abundantly. Avoid hydraulic lifts which are almost universally terrifying to anyone with a fear of falling.

Other safety/health concerns

While we're on the subject of safety, here are some other quick tips:

- If possible, eliminate the possibility of scalding water by setting the water heater at 120 or 122 degrees F. People in the late stages of AD seem particularly vulnerable to extremes of temperature. They may require cooler water than we would find comfortable.

- Place everything you will need for bathing and dressing the person in the bathroom before bringing him in so you will not need to leave him alone once the bath/shower is begun.

- If a person has arthritis, osteoporosis or another painful condition, it's important to give her pain medication and make sure it has taken effect before starting her bath. Transfer her gently into and out of the shower or tub. Wash her; don't scrub her. Pat her dry; don't rub her dry. Tell her what you're going to do before each step so she is not startled by your touch. Acknowledge her painful condition and apologize for any discomfort you cause. (A research study on nurses who were most effective in giving inoculations showed that those who acknowledged that the shot might hurt were considered the gentlest.)

- Use bath time to examine the person's body for redness, bruising, rashes and skin tears. If he is diabetic, examine his feet and be sure to wash and dry them carefully. Many large-breasted women develop skin rashes under their bosoms. A thin layer of cornstarch (which is less expensive and more absorbent than baby powder) can prevent and cure rashes here or in other folds of the skin. Incontinent people who develop rashes on their buttocks can often be helped with A&D ointment. Alert your doctor or nurse to anything unusual.

- Move out of range any electrical appliances or glass bottles which could be pulled into the tub or shower.

- If you have washed the person's hair, dry it completely to prevent a chill.

- Use a non-slip bathmat and wipe up puddles caused by dripping water.

- Many people in the later stages of AD require the aid of two people to transfer them in and out of a tub or shower. Don't risk causing bruises, abrasions or a fall by trying to do it alone.

- Grab bars are intended primarily as entering and exiting aids. The person who clings desperately to a grab bar while being bathed is usually afraid of the water or afraid of falling. He probably needs to be bathed in a seated position. Then if he is still fearful, try asking for his assistance in holding the washcloth, shampoo bottle, or that rubber ducky.

- For most people with AD, a hand-held shower is preferable to an overhead shower. The hand-held version enables you to get a person used to the bathing process gently by starting at her feet as if she were walking into a pool. It also allows you (or her) to control

  Activities of daily living

the direction of the spray away from her head and hair, if that is a concern – which it often is.

Make bathing a nurturing experience

The key, as in everything else, is **flexibility**. First, recognize that as people age, they sweat less, and their skin becomes drier. That means **daily bathing is usually not necessary or even desirable**. A bath once or twice a week and regular sponge bathing of hands, faces, underarms and the genital area is often sufficient. Begin by setting reasonable goals. Then look for ways to accomplish them. My favorite innovative caregiver was the woman who found she could bathe one third of her husband while he was sleeping before he would awaken and resist, so every third night he had the equivalent of one whole bath!

Take your concern for the person's comfort a step further. **Pamper her.**

- Make sure the room is warm enough for the person who is undressed and often a passive participant. Bathroom heaters in the wall or ceiling can help lessen the disparity between the room temperature and the water temperature. Use heated towel racks (or an in-room microwave or clothes dryer to heat the towels).

- Use terry cloth bathrobes, bath sheets or beach towels for after-bath warming up and drying. We are all irritated by the too-skimpy towels common to certain motel chains. Feet grow cold quickly on a linoleum or tile floor, so look for ways to cover them up, too.

- Learn her favorite soap scents and preferred shampoo and conditioner and use them.

- Follow baths with soothing scented-lotion massages to faces, hands, arms, feet and legs which are often badly in need of moisturizing.

- For people who don't like bathing, help them find pleasure in its finish by offering them hot chocolate or a backrub.

- Also look for pleasant ways to partially bathe residents. Smelly feet are often both cured and soothed with a warm, Epsom salts foot bath.

In short, let familiarity breed contentment.

Consultant Joanne Rader is widely recognized for changing how the disabled elderly are bathed. See Resources for more information.

7—Nutrition and Hydration

All people are made alike.
They are made of bones, flesh and dinners.
Only the dinners are different.
—Gertrude Cheney (written in 1927 at age 9)

A huge aspect of quality caregiving is providing healthy meals and adequate hydration, but since our dinners are indeed very different – meaning our personal preferences as to what, where and when we eat – that isn't easy. This chapter is focused on practical suggestions for improving the nutrition and hydration of people with Alzheimer's disease in the early through middle stages. Very late in the disease process people with dementia tend to have much more difficulty with swallowing. While there is still much that can be done at that point, the decisions about what to do and how to do it should be made under the care of a physician and dietitian. Furthermore, many people with dementia have other health concerns which means they may need special diets. This chapter makes no attempt to address those issues, but does provide insights into making mealtimes the pleasurable events we always want them to be.

Create context and setting

To encourage optimal eating and drinking, there are two main rules: create a pleasant atmosphere and provide healthy, appetizing food and beverages. When people with Alzheimer's disease begin to lose their ability to eat independently, it is often the former rule that is more important than the second.

Creating the pleasant atmosphere begins well before the meal. For example, if people have just participated in a program of exercise, dance or sport, it may take them awhile to calm down and prepare their minds for eating. Some people suggest that for the evening meal it is a good idea to begin with a late afternoon program of calm, such as a vesper service if you are part of a faith community or simply soothing music or a few minutes rocking on the porch and watching the birds at the feeder.

For centuries, the Japanese have been famous for their highly ritualized tea ceremony that incorporates the four elements of harmony, respect, purity and tranquility. One author described the effect like this: "We listen quietly to the boiling water in the kettle, which sounds like a breeze passing through the pine needles, and become oblivious of all worldly woes and worries . . . " (*Zen and Japanese Culture*) Those elements permeate the entire meal and leave participants with both a pleasingly full stomach and a brimming spirit to enhance the hours that follow.

Perhaps that tranquility is an impossible ideal in our everyday lives, but the point is, setting the mood counts. Yes, healthy food matters, but as J. Robbins said in *Diet for a New America:*

Those who eat beer and franks
With cheer and thanks,
Will be healthier than those who eat
Sprouts and bread with doubts and dread.

Hydration

Reasons for dehydration

We have all heard that for optimum health we need to drink 6-8 glasses (48 - 64 ounces) of water or other healthy liquids a day. In very cold weather when furnaces dry the indoor air or in hot weather, the total ounces should increase. You may also have heard that when you drink alcohol or caffeine, you have to add an equivalent amount of water

  Activities of daily living

to the total, since those substances deplete us. The bottom line is, it's not easy for most of us to drink all the water we should, and for people with dementia, there are a number of other factors that may interfere with their intake:

- **Illness or infections**. When we don't feel well, we often find it too much effort to get our own juice or water. When someone else is caring for us, we sometimes don't ask for what we need, because we "don't want to be a bother." Bladder infections which make urination painful may cause some people to stop drinking with the hope that they will need to urinate less, even though that may actually prolong the infection.

- **Medications**. Some medications have a side effect of being diuretic even if that is not the purpose for which they are being taken. The person with dementia (or his caregiver) may fail to understand the need for additional liquids to replace what is being lost, especially if going to the bathroom "too often" is perceived as a problem. Other medications increase befuddlement thereby interfering with a person's ability to pour her own drinks, ask for water, or get to the bathroom in time.

- People with dementia may **have agnosia**, the inability to recognize once familiar objects. Thus, they won't perceive that a water pitcher or a tea pot could relieve their thirst. Water pitchers next to bedsides in nursing homes are almost universally recognized as ineffective for people with dementia. By the time people with AD need a nursing home, they no longer understand the meaning of the water pitcher.

- The natural progression of dementia also involves **apraxia**, meaning the inability to initiate and carry out previously learned tasks. People may have problems in sequencing actions or they may know what to do, but cannot follow through with the necessary motor movements. They may recognize the pitcher as a source of liquid, but don't know how to pour themselves a glass of water.

- People with dementia may also **lose verbal skills.** It may seem a simple matter to tell someone, *I'm thirsty,* but for the person with Alzheimer's disease, it's often no longer in his vocabulary. In fact, as I noted in the companion book, *Alzheimer's Basic Caregiving,* a person who has a "pat" answer for all occasions may answer the question, *Are you thirsty?* with the phrase, *No thank you, dear, I'm fine,* regardless of her needs. Nor is a person's behavior recognized as a plea for drink, although many people who seem to be walking about aimlessly may, in fact, be thirsty.

So what's the big deal?

Since most people probably don't consciously drink all the liquids they should each day, you might ask, what's the harm? The answer is, most of us have enough presence of mind to drink when we are thirsty, so if we don't drink enough to give ourselves the world's softest skin, we also aren't at risk for drinking so little that we become delirious. However, a person with dementia may not recognize his own thirst and may not be able to meet the need even when he does. He is at risk for all of the following:

- Incontinence and bladder infections due to concentrated urine that irritates the urinary tract
- Constipation and bowel obstruction
- Loss of appetite from dry mouth (Saliva tends to decrease with age.)
- Dry, itchy skin
- Low blood pressure
- Dizziness and increased falls
- Nausea
- Heart problems

  Activities of daily living

- Poor wound healing
- Confusion / delirium
- Pneumonia

   So it *is* a big deal.

What can we do?

The basic answer is simple: **Offer lots of little drinks often.** If you give me a big glass of orange juice in the morning (92% water), I might not get it all down, but if you give me 4 ounces of juice with my toast and I have a bowl of cream of wheat (90% water) or oatmeal (80% water), and then you give me some decaf coffee while we sit and read the newspaper's gossip column, I will be off to a good start.

Another 4 ounces of apple juice (88% water) before we start our exercises, a cup of fruited yogurt (71% water) after we finish, and 4 ounces of water to "wet our whistles" before a sing-along and slowly we are getting all the liquid we need – and enjoying it as part of a social occasion as well. Many have found that the social context is a key element in increasing food and beverage intake. Other ideas include:

- a decaf coffee klatch
- twice daily juice breaks
- afternoon tea
- a soda shop set-up that serves orange sherbet blended in milk
- a lemonade stand in the garden

   Use your imagination. Brainstorm solutions.

When we were kids we were told that drinking our milk before our meal would spoil our appetite. Now many nutritionists encourage a small glass of liquid – water, cranberry juice or non-alcoholic wine, for example – to *stimulate* the appetite of people with dementia, so it's worth a try. Others have found that people tend to eat and drink more when they participate in a "Happy Hour" setting: Serve healthy appetizers and not-too-sweet drinks. (Milk and citrus drinks can produce extra mucous in the throat and are therefore inappropriate for some people.) Alcohol, as noted earlier, increases dehydration, but for many people a couple of ounces of wine may be more boon than bane. That is something for you and your doctor to decide.

The key is not to simply offer water and other beverages, but to make sure the person drinks them. You may have to increase the trips to the bathroom with this person, but that's preferable to a bladder infection or delirium from too little liquid.

Nutrition

Scents and taste in AD

Most people begin to experience a decline in their ability to smell at about age 60. As they age, they may have difficulty distinguishing between smells and require higher concentrations to detect an odor. However, people with Alzheimer's disease tend to experience a more profound loss of smell, and it often precedes losses in vision and hearing. Some experts believe that this early and striking alteration is even a reliable precursor to AD.

It used to be thought that the number of taste buds also diminished as we age, but according to the Wisconsin Dental Association, research belies that myth. It is true, however, that more than half of our taste sensations are dependent on our sense of smell; therefore, it is logical to think that as our sense of smell diminishes, so does our sense of taste. In addition, most older adults take multiple medications, many of which interfere with taste. Furthermore, in residential care settings, medical smells such as alcohol and cleaning smells such as ammonia may contribute to a distorted sense of taste and suppress appetites. The bottom line? People with AD may tolerate and even crave spicier, more flavorful foods than you might think.

Progression-related challenges

In the early to middle stages, people with AD who are living independently may become malnourished because:

- They have forgotten the steps involved in shopping for groceries, following a recipe or preparing a meal.
- They may be unable to safely operate a stove and may no longer remember how to operate a microwave.
- They may be unable to recognize when food is spoiled or rancid. Comedian Rita Rudner has a line: *My husband thinks health food is anything he eats before the expiration date.* In her context it is funny. But people with dementia often can't smell when food has gone bad, can't find the expiration date on the package (which is often printed too small for their eyes to read) and would find it meaningless in any case because they don't know today's date.
- They may have trouble reading the small print directions on packaged food, and following the directions they *can* read.
- The packaging itself – cardboard cartons, air-tight pouches, plastic film – may mystify them.

Consequently, they may subsist on crackers or other foods that require no preparation. Malnutrition aggravates signs of dementia and increases risk of infection and other health problems.

People in the early to middle stages of Alzheimer's disease living in a residential care setting do not have these food preparation challenges, but they can easily become anxious or agitated if:

- Their meal is different from their neighbor's;

- The behavior of the person seated next to them is upsetting; or
- There is too long a wait for their meal to be served. (Although never good, this is especially aggravating at breakfast; try to at least provide coffee, juice or a piece of fruit. Some people need a banana or piece of toast even before getting out of bed. At other mealtimes, provide at least an appetizer such as cheese and crackers – something to start out with.)

In later stages, they may become agitated if their dentures or clothing or continence care pads are causing discomfort.

As Alzheimer's disease progresses, many people develop "the guppy syndrome" – eating everything in sight with no apparent recognition of being satiated. They don't end up floating upside down and bloated in the fish bowl, but they may experience a weight gain, possibly because they often seem to have a particular fondness for sweets. Then as the disease progresses further, this is almost invariably followed by a weight loss, perhaps due to a disease-related change in metabolism.

Other challenges related to changes in their brains also arise. They may:

- Fail to understand the proper use of utensils, beginning with the knife, followed by the fork and eventually the spoon. (Misuse of the knife may show up when a person, like the Mother Goose character, tries to eat his peas with it, but it may also come about when he refuses meat, afraid to admit he can no longer cut it himself. In that case, help him by cutting it into bite-sized pieces before serving it to him.)
- Be unaware of their food and their reason for sitting there.

- Out of boredom and incomprehension, play with their food (pouring cranberry juice over their mashed potatoes and peas) or take food from others' plates. Understandably, this can be a turn-off to higher functioning diners.
- Fail to perceive food as food, or alternatively, perceive non-food items as edible.

The depression connection

As discussed in the companion book, *Alzheimer's Basic Caregiving,* people with dementia living on their own are often malnourished due to a combination of factors related to dementia and depression. Their dementia inhibits their ability to prepare healthy meals. They may be depressed for reasons ranging from their awareness of their memory impairment to the loss of a spouse or distance from other family members. People who are depressed are likely to have little appetite or little interest in eating alone, so they may become further malnourished. When people are malnourished, particularly when they have severe vitamin B deficiency, their symptoms of dementia and depression are aggravated. It becomes a vicious cycle, and it's soon difficult to tell which can first – the deficiency or the depression? Sometimes symptoms of dementia can be relieved simply by returning to a healthy diet, so recognizing how these three elements intertwine is essential to quality care. We know how to treat malnutrition and depression, and if treating them doesn't make the dementia disappear, it at least makes the person healthier.

However, knowing how to treat malnutrition and depression doesn't mean the solutions are easy. For example, Meals on Wheels is a wonderful organization for helping people to get the pre-prepared food they need, but some people resist their services. Anti-depressants have helped millions of people, but people with dementia often need assistance in remembering to take those and other medications. You will meet obstacles and will need persistence to overcome them.

Make it homey

People with Alzheimer's disease may take an hour or more to eat as their disease progresses, so the number one rule for caregivers is to remain patient and relaxed. Stay attuned and offer assistance and encouragement as needed. Creating a comfortable atmosphere is as important to digestion as the food itself, and often that atmosphere is more dependent on emotional factors than physical ones. I once had lunch in a Thai restaurant where all customers were given a card that said in part: *No matter what we eat, a stressed physiology will not make the best of it.* The card urged us to refuse only one guest at our table: *Never entertain negativity.*

To create a pleasing physical atmosphere, consider your best memories of family gatherings around the kitchen or dining room table. What were the elements that made it memorable? Usually the answer has to do with good smells, good food and people who love each other. My guess is there wasn't a nurse passing out medications, or dining aides shouting across the room at one another or a person scraping garbage and stacking dirty dishes onto a cart behind our heads. We can't always recreate home, but here are the elements that we know to be helpful:

- **Quiet.** People with Alzheimer's disease cannot filter out irrelevant information, so a noisy room provides many distractions that interfere with their ability to concentrate on eating, and often produces frequent startle responses. You can decrease noise levels with multiple soft surfaces such as tablecloths or cloth placemats, upholstered chairs, curtains or fabric wall hangings (quilts work well), and carpeted floors (consider carpeting the walls, too, to a chair-rail height).

- **Smaller spaces.** Many people with AD are more comfortable in normal-sized dining rooms. Cavernous halls are often overwhelming and filled with loud echoes. In residential care settings, if separate dining rooms serving 4 – 8 people are not feasible daily, try to offer luncheons for a specially selected small group at least weekly, or try dividing up the dining room with screens or other artificial spacers. Also recognize that some people, especially if they have lived alone for a long time or have a tendency to spill or dribble their food, prefer to eat alone. The desire to dine in the privacy of one's room is not necessarily anti-social behavior.

- **Contrasts.** Tabletops should provide a contrast to the floor. Plates should be a contrasting color to tabletops or tablecloths and placemats or at least have a contrasting edge. Contrasts are provided by differences in intensity, not simply color. White and black provide strong contrasts, but royal blue and purple may not be distinguishable to very old eyes. Contrasting placemats can help define territory in a group setting. Try to avoid putting pale foods on a white plate (mashed potatoes, rice, cauliflower, chicken). Watch for individual color preferences, and avoid china with flower and fruit patterns which may be perceived as food.

- **Adequate lighting.** Wall sconces may provide atmosphere, but not enough illumination to see one's food clearly. On the other hand, some windows and overhead lights produce an upsetting glare that can also be reflected on smooth tabletops if tablecloths are not used.

- **Elimination of clutter.** As their disease progresses, table settings for people with AD should be kept simple. Put out only the dishes and utensils which are necessary for the meal or which you know a particular person can use handily. Flowers or other centerpieces, sugar packet containers and extra bread plates, for example, are likely to provide distractions rather than pleasing elegance. In residential care settings, the dining room itself may appear cluttered to the person intimidated by large spaces filled with many tables and chairs, particularly if they are close together or if one must also navigate around wheelchairs and walkers. A person who hesitates at a dining room door is often sending a message of discomfort with the space. Many people with Alzheimer's disease do better seated around a normal home-sized dining room table and eating family style, with no more than 6 or 8 people in the room. For others, clutter may be represented not by people or tables and chairs, but by a plateful of too many foods in too large proportions.

Make it a social occasion

As noted earlier in this chapter, appetites can be stimulated by emphasizing the social context of the meal. Many people enjoy helping with meal preparation such as chopping vegetables, slicing cheese or setting the table, particularly if the standards for success are not set too high. (For example, does the napkin have to be left of the plate, the spoon to the right?) This is an area calling for creativity in building on the strengths of the people involved. Sometimes it's a matter of breaking things down into simple steps. A person who can't measure ingredients may be surprisingly adept at chopping or stirring them. One author in *Food, Glorious Food* described a man who could not cut up the apples for the fruit salad but who proved a master at polishing them. Another author in the same book described a one-on one baking activity with a woman named Annie, who when the mixing bowl was on the table, found it hard to participate.

The author put a towel in Annie's lap to protect her clothing, placed the bowl on top of the towel, and although Annie occasionally came close to losing her grip, she successfully mixed the ingredients in a way she had probably done hundreds of times before. Things won't get done quickly this way and they may not get done perfectly, but the real goal is participants enjoying the process, setting the tone for a pleasant meal.

Food preparation is another area where aromas are worth a try. (If the people with AD can't smell them, they are at least likely to be stimulated by the caregivers who are talking about and enjoying the smells.) Perking coffee and frying bacon are wonderful get-out-of-bed smells, and is there any reason that toast can't be prepared in the dining room where it's eaten? Some people have found success in drawing people to a room where something aromatic is simmering in a crock pot. Try onion soup, lemon or orange extract, ginger, tomato or garlic. Baking bread or brownies or popping popcorn always creates a festive feeling and wonderful fragrances. Peering into the crock pot or listening to popcorn pop can also stir up old memories of great smells, even if the person can't smell them now. (Note: Popcorn is not a good food to serve to people with swallowing difficulties or who choke easily.)

You can also stimulate appetites by involving people with AD in meal or party planning. Look through recipe books with inviting pictures. Talk about favorite foods and recipes. Plan the events around the party – invitations, decorations, games, music, etc.

Creating pleasant conversation during meals seems like a good idea and sometimes is, but be aware that as their disease progresses, many people need every bit of concentration they can muster for eating. Then conversation is a distraction, although you may find you can take a break now and then and perhaps talk between courses. Also be sure that people seated together have been introduced to each other. They may not remember the names, but they are likely to realize introductions are a part of being polite.

The need to concentrate is also one reason background music may be a detriment to optimal eating. It can also interfere with normal conversation if a person has a hearing deficit. (Others have found success with it.)

Social occasions are likely to be enhanced if people of like abilities are seated together. A person who can still eat well independently may lose her appetite and feel demeaned if seated next to a person who requires much more assistance.

Social occasions are also enhanced if the procedure is familiar. Some people have had success in serving meals family style at the table rather than being handed a plate already filled with food. Others have found that restaurant style – with linen tablecloths and nice china – provides an atmosphere for people to rise to, and that frequently they do.

Positioning

How easily people eat and how much they eat can also have a great deal to do with the position of their bodies. Many older women have osteoporosis that causes them to hunch over and can interfere with both their breathing and their ability to eat. Sitting in a wheel chair for long periods is uncomfortable. To eat, the person should be transferred to a regular chair. Centering a person's torso above the hips improves her balance and stability. Seating them with their feet comfortably on the floor in front of them helps them feel supported and grounded. Others may need their head, elbows or other body parts supported by pillows or rolled towels to keep them in a good position for swallowing.

  Activities of daily living

It is especially important for people to be as upright as possible when they eat, perhaps even tilted slightly forward. The person's head should not tilt backward while eating or drinking as this increases the risk of choking. Indeed, at least one dietitian notes that prolonged craning of the neck is uncomfortable and may pinch tiny capillaries in the neck, temporarily halting blood supply. In an older person, this may cause momentary unconsciousness and lead to a fall. Chairs with arms and high backs can often help with positioning and provide greater support.

Consult a physical or occupational therapist for more ideas if you are caring for someone for whom positioning is a particular challenge.

Other tricks and tips

Some dietitians suggest using small servings and small plates to help a person feel less overwhelmed by quantities of food. For those who have forgotten they ate an hour ago – or who, in fact, refused to – a small plate is also handy for reheating a serving in the microwave. Avoid overloading the china. Using a small bowl and filling it to the rim with fruit salad is still intimidating and makes the fruit difficult to spear.

For some people, three foods on a plate represent a deluge of choices. They do better if each food is served separately in a small bowl and offered one at a time. Other people do better with five or six small meals throughout the day. Here are other hints:

- Plastic cups and mugs tend to make less noise, are unbreakable and easier for some persons to handle, but try to serve everyone at the meal with similar "china," even if it's plastic. Some people are acutely aware when their plates and cups are different. Avoid plastic utensils as these break easily and can be dangerous.

- Paper or Styrofoam cups are easy to tip, and Styrofoam is thought by more than a few people with AD to be crunchy and good to eat, so avoid using those, too. Some people in the later stages may try to eat paper napkins; if that becomes a problem, try cloth ones.
- Putting a damp cloth under a plate will keep it from sliding on a smooth surface.
- Using bowls or plates with one high edge help people to get their food onto a fork more easily.
- Some people have found that weighted or specially curved utensils are helpful, but experimentation may be necessary, as others will reject these unfamiliar tools. Also recognize that initial rejection does not mean the person with AD will not get used to and benefit from these innovations over a period of weeks or months.

Helping the person who isn't a self-starter

If a person seated at a table does not immediately begin eating when food is placed in front of him, try to determine the reason. In residential care settings, some people may be waiting for the group to say grace. Others may be worried about paying for the meal. Some people may be reassured by noting that it is covered by insurance or Medicare (they don't usually accept the idea that it is free), and others have found that creating meal cards to be punched works well. Others may be waiting for a family member to join them; they may be mollified by an empty chair set beside them to "save a place" for the relative.

Some people may not like where they are seated. People who are between a wall and a table may feel trapped. (Try angling the tables in the room.) People who are easily distracted may need to face a wall to limit their vision of other diners. Others may be upset when another person sits in "their" place. Usually the usurper is trying to do the best she can and may not know she has offended anyone. One

  Activities of daily living

creative assisted living residence solved this challenge by telling the person that there was a space reserved for her "in first class." The woman willingly moved to the "upgraded area." Others "reserve" a person's place by putting her sweater over the chair back.

Some people worry about embarrassing themselves by spilling their food on their clothes. I have a personal prejudice against bibs, but will accept aprons which were left on after assisting with food preparation or napkins tucked into one's blouse, as I see those as adult solutions. Sometimes it's a simple matter of positioning a person closer to the table and more upright.

Others may have little interest in eating when they are overtired. Experts suggest that people with AD should have their main meal at noon when their energy levels are likely to be highest. It is not unusual for someone to be able to eat toast and scrambled eggs for breakfast and manage reasonably well, but by evening that same person may not seem to know how to pick up a fork and use it. Pay attention to the person's abilities and how they change over the day.

Other people, as suggested earlier, have problems with packaging – they can't open a milk carton or cream container or peel a banana or tangerine.

When more cueing is required, here are some ideas:

- Some people can be helped by gently expressed verbal cues offered one at a time. Begin by calling the person by name, recognizing you may have to do so several times before getting her attention. Then give directions: *Sit here . . . Pick up your fork . . . Try the beans . . . Would you like some apple juice?*

- Others may require a combination of cues, such as actually handing the fork to the person and saying, *Use this for your mashed potatoes.*

- Still others may require a jump start, i.e., helping with the first bite by feeding the person with your hand over his hand holding the fork or spoon.
- Some persons need periodic jump starts. They can remember to eat for a few bites and then they put down their fork, forget why they are sitting there and need to be cued all over again.
- Others need to be fed from start to finish and may need to be told with each bite: *Open your mouth, Mary. . . Close your lips, Mary . . . Chew, Mary . . . Swallow.*

Look for solvable conditions

Often eating difficulties are caused by solvable conditions that the person with dementia simply can't articulate, such as:

- Pain – from arthritis, poorly fitting dentures or food caught beneath dentures, headache, stomachache, even shoes that are too tight. Pain is always distracting.
- Visual problems – The person may not be able to see her food clearly. Can you help her understand what she has been served and where it is on her plate? Is she wearing glasses? Is the prescription for distance? Might she actually see better if they were removed while she ate?
- Room temperature – If a person is too hot or too cold, it is hard to concentrate on eating. Watch out for drafts caused by open windows, hallway breezes and being seated under air conditioning vents.
- Dislikes the food – Perhaps this person has always detested beets, or perhaps she simply finds the meal in front of her distasteful. What are her favorite foods? What does she consider a comfort food? Can you serve her those? (One informal survey found that chicken soup and toast far outstripped any others as comfort foods for

  Activities of daily living

older adults, but that was years ago. I suspect ice cream has risen closer to the top since then.)

Also watch for sudden changes in eating behavior that may indicate infection, illness or some other condition requiring attention. A change in ability that persists often indicates a person is transitioning and will continue to need a higher level of assistance.

Finger foods

Many people whose skill with a knife and fork has severely diminished can still manage to eat independently if they are given finger foods. Finger foods are also a good solution for the small percentage of people with dementia who seem to have a strong need to keep moving and who need their nourishment "on the run."

In the privacy of one's home, "finger foods" can be almost anything to a flexible caregiver. In a restaurant or residential care setting, greater discretion may be in order, but look, too, for innovative solutions. Encouraging finger foods has a purpose beyond self-feeding since some research suggests that there is a correlation between physical and mental exercise, which means that eating on one's own helps with mental alertness.

Most people tend to think of finger foods as hot dogs, hamburgers, pizza and French fries, but the choices can be far healthier and broader in scope. Chicken, shish-ka-bobs, quiche, fruit (bananas, grapes, slices of apples, oranges, pears, etc.) and vegetable slices (vegetables can be lightly steamed to soften them), cheese, dry cereal (Cheerios), boiled eggs and deviled eggs, represent just a beginning. Many people like sandwiches; for those who walk as they eat, grilled cheese and peanut butter work well, but the possibilities increase if you consider the healthy sandwiches which can be made with pocket pita bread. Also think beyond pepperoni to fresh tomatoes, spinach, zucchini, broccoli and any other vegetable as a pizza topping. Serve pancakes with a light coating of jam or peanut butter wound up like a jelly roll. Soups, of course, can be served in mugs.

People who do not yet need finger foods may just need foods easy to get onto a spoon – scrambled eggs, applesauce, cottage cheese, casseroles. Aim for a consistency of textures. Vegetables in a thin broth are much more likely to cause choking than vegetables in a casserole or even a cream soup. On the other hand, to stimulate the palate try a grainy texture like toast – it's a great wake-up food.

Look beyond the obvious

Encouraging people to eat well sometimes requires looking beyond the obvious. One woman in an assisted living community refused to sit down to eat. By questioning her family, staff learned that the woman had worked as a kitchen aide all her life and had always eaten standing up on the run; when staff allowed her to do so, she continued to eat well. Mothers of large families may have had similar life experiences.

You may also get better results by experimenting with food temperatures. Some experts have noticed a decreased tolerance in people with AD to extremes of hot and cold foods and beverages, so that serving items closer to body temperature rather than normal serving temperature works better. Another expert noted that the sense of different tastes (sweet, salt, bitter) are best perceived at body temperature and that people will be more aware of flavors if food is served at body temperature. Others, of course, find heated liquids such as hot chocolate or a cup of tea good for warming up both body and soul. Cold fluids tend to elicit a cough reflex.

Also never overlook people's personal preferences. One woman was assessed for her eating independence by being given green beans, and as she did nothing with them was deemed to need someone to hand feed her. Another nutritionist came along and assessed her abilities with apple pie and found her fully independent.

Some personal preferences are based on what foods do to their bodies. Some people resist oranges because their acidic qualities trouble the stomach; others resist milk products because they increase the mucous in their throats; others resist vegetables that give them gas. (Adding caraway can overcome that problem.) Some people have trouble swallowing sticky foods like peanut butter, and others resist chips and crunchy foods that make them choke easily.

People who were raised with certain ethnic foods as their staples can often have their appetites stimulated by a return to what is familiar.

On the other hand, you might be surprised by people's willingness to try something new. *Our chef is trying out a new recipe and would like your opinion.* People with dementia remain curious and want to be useful. If you are a family caregiver, just vary the line: *I'm thinking of submitting this recipe to the United Way cookbook fundraiser. Do you think it's good enough?*

End stage issues

At some point in the course of their progressive condition, a person with Alzheimer's disease will stop eating and can no longer be hand fed. I personally do not believe in tube-feeding people with dementia and see it as cruel and futile. We can postpone death, but we cannot prevent it. When a person is no longer able to eat or drink, death is near and should be welcomed. It is the natural way people have died for millions of years. For many people, this issue is not as clear-cut, and because this book is primarily focused on people with Alzheimer's disease who are years away from death, I do not want to belabor the point here. However, if this is a topic of interest to you, I know of no better resource than the 80-page booklet, *Hard Choices for Loving People*, by Hank Dunn, a former Hospice chaplain with whom I once served on the board of directors of the Northern Virginia Alzheimer's Chapter. See the Bibliography for details

Activities of daily living

A Final Message to Caregivers

A few years ago, my daughter and I had the tremendous experience of riding mules deep into the Grand Canyon from the North Rim. The mule team leader, easily seeing my inexperience, assigned me to a mule named Maude, a gentle creature who chose her own pace. She was particularly immune to prodding on the return, uphill trip, and I soon stopped caring that I was causing the last three mules to lag behind. But that's when I also learned she had been misnamed. To put this as delicately as possible, she ought to have been named Tooter. She was not in the least discreet – indeed, there were times when she sounded like a trumpet in a John Phillips Sousa marching band. The mule path was also shared by hikers, and she startled quite a few of the adults. Children found her hilarious, of course. (Frankly, so did I.) One hiker thought she might be pregnant. She was momentarily quiet as we passed, so I didn't enlighten him to the true cause of her distended belly. However, when we finally returned to the stables, she gave a whole new meaning to "running out of gas."

The young woman on the mule behind mine showed infinite patience (but tended to keep her distance) at one point saying, *Whatever gets her up the hill.* The life of a caregiver is often stressful. Any caregiving book worth its salt will admonish caregivers to take good care of themselves: eat a balanced diet, get enough sleep, exercise regularly, surround yourself with cheerful friends and keep a positive attitude. But the reality is that sometimes caregiving is a steep journey with a heavy load. Sometimes the unhealthy comfort food or the foregone exercise class is what gets us up the day's hill. Remember Maude, set your own pace, and make no excuses.

Resources

R esources
This book is based on the advice I provided in my newsletter *Wiser Now*, which was published from 1992 – 1999. My first mentor (and friend) in the field was Mary Lucero who is president of Geriatric Resources, Inc. (800-359-0390,   ). Much of what I wrote in the early years was based on interviewing her about particular topics, and I am forever grateful for her kindness in sharing. Over the years I came to know many experts. I also attended conferences, read journals, others' newsletters and every book I could find on Alzheimer's disease. I cannot provide precise footnotes for how I learned everything I learned, in part because a lot of similar advice can be found in multiple resources, but following are the sources for each chapter that are easily referenced. Also see the Bibliography.

Chapter 2: Dressing

Speaking Our Minds by Lisa Snyder is referenced in the Bibiliography.

Some sources for Adaptive Clothing:

- Buck & Buck: www.buckandbuck.com or 800-458-0600
- Comfort Clothing: www.comfortclothing.com or 888-640-0814
- Easy Does It ™: www.myeasydoesit.com
- MJ Designs: www.mjdesignsinc.com or 800-722-2021
- Silverts: www.silverts.com or 800-387-7088
- Wardrobe Wagon: www.wardrobewagon.com or 800-992-2737

Chapter 3: Grooming

The foreign translations are from *The Best of Uncle John's Bathroom Reader*, Bathroom Reader's Press, Ashland, OR, 1995. ISBN 1-879682-62-1

Chapter 4: Oral Hygiene

As noted, my primary sources for this chapter were the websites for the Mayo Clinic (www.MayoClinic.com), Colgate (www.colgate.com) and the Wisconsin Dental Association (www.wda.org.)

Chapter 6: Bathing

The person who is considered one of the foremost experts and compassionate crusaders for bathing reform in long-term care settings, especially among people with dementia is Joanne Rader, whose work can be found at www.bathingwithoutabattle.unc.edu. This is also a source for the video *Bathing Without a Battle* available for $30 plus shipping. Another reference which could prove helpful on this topic is: Barrick, A.L., Rader, J., Hoeffer, B., Sloane, P.,(Ed). "Bathing without a battle: Personal care for persons with dementia," New York , Springer Publishering Company.

Chapter 7: Nutrition and Hydration

Although ideas for this chapter came from many sources, my two favorite books on this topic are *Bon Appetit! The Joy of Dining in Long-Term Care* by Jitka Zgola and Gilbert Bordillon and *Food, Glorious Food, Perspectives on food and dementia* edited by Mary Marshall. See Bibliography.

B ibliography

This book and its companion, *Alzheimer's Basic Caregiving – an ABC Guide*, are intended to provide useful advice in a palatable style. My goal is to be brief and practical, but it requires me to leave unsaid much that I might want to add. For greater detail I invite you to turn to others. The following books, listed in alphabetical order by author are among my favorite resources. Most of them have been written by people I am honored to call my friends. That means they were chosen with a bias, but I choose my friends in this field carefully – these are not the only outstanding people committed to quality care for people with Alzheimer's disease, but they are some of the best and the nicest, and their advice is wise.

Bell, Virginia and Troxel, David. *The Best Friends Approach to Alzheimer's Care*. Baltimore: Health Professions Press. © 1996. ISBN 1878812351. Virginia and David have written several "Best Friends" volumes since the first one in 1996 and I recommend them all. Their books are reader-friendly and were the first I found to take a positive attitude toward Alzheimer's disease, illustrating the fun and good times that are still possible after diagnosis.

Brawley, Elizabeth C. *Design Innovations for Aging and Alzheimer's*. New York: John Wiley & Sons, Inc. © 2005. ISBN 0471681180. This book and Betsy's previous book for Wiley (*Designing for Alzheimer's Disease: Strategies for Creating Better Care Environments* © 1997. ISBN 0471139203) are, in my opinion, the penultimate books for designing residential care settings, but also provide insights for families looking for residential care.

Dunn, Hank. *Hard Choices for Loving People: CPR, Artificial Feeding, Comfort Care and the Patient with a Life-Threatening Illness*. A&A Publishers, Inc. © 2001. ISBN 1928560032. This inexpensive publication is available through Amazon and other book dealers, but the easiest way to order is by calling 703-707-0169 (voice mail) or sending an email to AAPublish@aol.com. This excellent resource is available in quantity at very low prices making it a great resource for group discussions or for handing out to patients, clients, resident families, etc. (www.hardchoices.com)

Fazio, Sam; Seman, Dorothy and Stansell, Jane. *Rethinking Alzheimer's Care.* Baltimore: Health Professions Press. © 1999. ISBN 1878812629. I admire all three of these authors, but Dorothy Seman will always have a special place in my heart and has been my moral compass throughout my journey into this disease.

Gwyther, Lisa. *Caring for People with Alzheimer's Disease: A Manual for Facility Staff.* © 2001. ISBN 0-9705219-3-6. This book was most recently updated in 2001, but is currently unavailable. However, you can check out others written by Lisa and other members of her staff by contacting the Duke Family Support Program at 919-660-7510 or through their website: www.geri.duke.edu.

Hellen, Carly. *Alzheimer's Disease: Activity-Focused Care, 2nd edition.* Boston: Butterworth-Heinemann Press. © 1998. ISBN 0750699086. Carly was an early guru in the field of Alzheimer's care, and as an occupational therapist (See also Carol Sifton and Jitka Zgola below) an author who is creative and practical in solving caregiving conundrums.

Henderson, Cary Smith. *Partial View: An Alzheimer's Journal.* Dallas: Southern Methodist University Press. © 1998. ISBN 0870744380. This book is one of the most reader friendly books written from the viewpoint of the person with AD because it consists of brief excerpts from his tape-recorded commentary on what it feels like to have Alzheimer's disease, and lots of striking photographs. The insights are priceless.

Kitwood, Tom. *Dementia Reconsidered: the Person Comes First.* Philadelphia: Open University Press. © 1997. ISBN 0335198554. Tom Kitwood is widely credited with inventing the concept of "person-centered care" and was certainly a pioneer in recognizing the remaining strengths in people with AD and the logic behind their behavior.

Kuhn, Daniel. *Alzheimer's Early Stages: First Steps for Family, Friends and Caregivers. (2nd edition).* Alameda, CA: Hunter House Publications. © 2003. ISBN 0897933974. It's telling that David Schenk, author of *The Forgetting*, quotes Dan's book extensively. Schenk's book is more commercially popular, but Dan's book is more worthy of reading.

Marshall, Mary, ed. *Food, Glorious Food, Perspectives on food and dementia.* Hawker Publications, London. © 2003. ISBN 187479071X. Because this is an English publication, it is a bit more difficult to get than the others listed here, but it's a lovely book.

Oliver, Rose and Bock, Francis A. *Coping with Alzheimer's: A Caregiver's Emotional Survival Guide.* North Hollywood, CA: Wilshire Book Company. © 1989. ISBN 0879804246. The first edition of this book is now almost 20 years old, but I know of no better book for caregivers who are battling their personal demons of guilt, anger, resentment, embarrassment, self-pity and overall stress.

Robinson, Anne; Spencer, Beth and White, Laurie. *Understanding Difficult Behaviors: Some Practical Suggestions for Coping with Alzheimer's Disease and Related Illnesses.* This book was originally published in the 1980s and even the most recent edition is about 10 years old. "Difficult Behaviors" is a term that is abhorrent to me because it suggests the person IS a problem rather than a person HAS a problem, but aside from the title, this is an excellent resource that has withstood the test of time. The easiest way to obtain this book is through an Alzheimer's chapter. One that carries it is Massachusetts: www.alzmass.org/publications.

Sifton, Carol Bowlby. *Navigating the Alzheimer's Journey: A Compass for Caregiving.* Baltimore: Health Professions Press. © 2004. ISBN 1932529047. In many ways Carol's book is a longer, more detailed book covering the topics I have tried to condense in mine. She writes from both personal and professional experience, telling useful stories and conducting thorough research before offering advice.

Snyder, Lisa. *Speaking Our Minds: Personal Reflections from Individuals with Alzheimer's.* New York: W.H. Freeman. © 2000. ISBN 0716740109. Lisa Snyder is a clinical social worker who has been counseling families at the Alzheimer's Disease Research Center (UCSD) in San Diego for nearly 20 years. This book features interviews of seven people with Alzheimer's disease and Lisa's cogent interpretation of their comments.

Warner, Mark. *The Complete Guide to Alzheimer's-Proofing Your Home (Revised Edition).* West Lafayette, IN: Purdue University Press. © 2000. ISBN 1557532206. Like several other books in this list with "Alzheimer's" in the title, my only complaint about the book is that the focus is too narrow. Mark gives excellent advice – and extensive resource lists for the products he recommends – for modifying your home for people with many conditions, not just AD.

Zgola, Jitka. *Care That Works: A Relationship Approach to Persons with Dementia.* Baltimore: Johns Hopkins University Press. © 1999. ISBN 0801860261. I can't say enough good things about the compassion with which Jitka writes and the amazing ideas that only occupational therapists seem to have at their fingertips.

Zgola, Jitka, Bordillon, Gilbert. *Bon Appetit! The Joy of Dining in Long-Term Care.* Baltimore: Health Professions Press. © 2001. ISBN 1878812688. This is a fabulous couple and they've written a fabulous book aimed at long-term care communities, but with ideas and recipes that can be helpful to families, too.

I have also made reference in this book and its companion, *Alzheimer's Basic Caregiving* to the video *Inside Looking Out.* This excellent video is available from Terra Nova Films (800-779-8491 or www. terranova.org)

About the author

Kathy Laurenhue, President of Wiser Now, Inc., has a master's degree in instructional technology (developing training) which she began to put to use in the field of elder care issues about 15 years ago after her parents' caregiving needs vastly increased. Her beloved mother died of Alzheimer's disease five years later and it was learning how to support her well-being that prompted much of Kathy's interest in dementia.

In more recent years she has focused on extensions of those original interests: brain aerobics for the stressed mind and life story sharing (learning to connect with one another). She is the author of *Getting to Know the Life Stories of Older Adults: Activities for Building Relationships* published by Health Professions Press (www.healthpropress.com, November 2006) and is currently writing a book tentatively titled *Getting to Know Your Brain*. Other publications are planned on caregiver cheer, creative training techniques and activities for dementia care.

Kathy also gives training seminars (for the public and as train-the-trainer workshops) on brain aerobics for the stressed mind, life story sharing, and sensitivity training for medical offices. She also writes a newsletter and activity ideas for www.activityconnection.com and online courses for www.caretrain.com. She can be reached by writing to Kathy@wisernow.com or calling 800-999-0795 (weekdays 9:00 – 5:00 Eastern time). Her website is www.wisernow.com.

Last, but certainly not least, she is the proud mother of two fabulous daughters and grandmother to two terrific grandchildren.

Notes

Notes

Notes

Notes

Notes